TRUE STORIES

From the

ATHLETIC TRAINING ROOM

TRUE STORIES
From the
ATHLETIC TRAINING ROOM

EDITED BY

KEITH M. GORSE, EdD, LAT, ATC
Assistant Professor and Clinical Coordinator
Department of Athletic Training
Duquesne University
Pittsburgh, Pennsylvania

FRANCIS FELD, DNP, CRNA, LAT, ATC, NRP
Staff CRNA, University of Pittsburgh Medical Center Passavant Hospital
Prehospital RN, Ross West View Emergency Medical Services
Supervisor, Allegheny County Hazmat Medical Team
Supervisory Nurse Specialist, PA-1 Disaster Medical Assistance Team
Pittsburgh, Pennsylvania

ROBERT O. BLANC, MS, LAT, ATC, EMT-P
Head Athletic Trainer—Football
Adjunct Clinical Instructor, Athletic Training Education Program
Duratz Athletic Facility, University of Pittsburgh
Pittsburgh, Pennsylvania

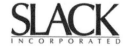

SLACK
INCORPORATED

www.Healio.com/books

ISBN: 978-1-63091-383-0

Published by: SLACK Incorporated
                  6900 Grove Road
                  Thorofare, NJ 08086 USA
                  Telephone: 856-848-1000
                  Fax: 856-848-6091
                  www.Healio.com/books

Contact SLACK Incorporated for more information about other books in this field or about the availability of our books from distributors outside the United States.

Library of Congress Cataloging-in-Publication Data

Names: Gorse, Keith M., editor. | Feld, Francis, editor. | Blanc, Robert O., editor.
Title: True stories from the athletic training room / edited by Keith M. Gorse, Francis Feld, Robert O. Blanc.
Description: Thorofare, NJ : SLACK Incorporated, [2018] | Includes bibliographical references and index.
Identifiers: LCCN 2017038484 (print) | LCCN 2017038963 (ebook) | ISBN 9781630913854 (Web) | ISBN 9781630913847 (epub) | ISBN 9781630913830 (alk. paper)
Subjects: | MESH: Athletic Injuries--diagnosis | Athletic Injuries--therapy | Sports Medicine--methods | Sports | Case Reports
Classification: LCC RD97 (ebook) | LCC RD97 (print) | NLM QT 261 | DDC 617.1/027--dc23

Last digit is print number: 10 9 8 7 6 5 4 3 2 1

DEDICATION

To all of the certified athletic trainers working at high schools, colleges, professional teams, industrial settings, sports medicine clinics, and wherever else. Their careers have been part of one big true story.

CONTENTS

ACKNOWLEDGMENTS

During the year that *True Stories From the Athletic Training Room* has been in production, many persons have assisted us. The staff at SLACK Incorporated was both supportive and patient during the entire process of developing this textbook. In particular, we would like to thank Mr. Brien Cummings and Mrs. Dani Malady, who provided the continuing support that gave us the initial okay to proceed and help make it happen.

We would like to thank the National Athletic Trainers' Association and all its members for allowing us to put together a comprehensive set of true stories that cover each of the 5 educational domains in athletic training.

Most importantly, we would like to thank all of our certified athletic trainers who contributed to this textbook, who openly shared their athletic training scenarios, which shaped this textbook in the way we wanted to have it presented to both certified and student athletic trainers, as well as anyone else interested in sports medicine for review and discussion.

LIST OF FIGURES

ABOUT THE EDITORS

Keith M. Gorse would like to thank all of the certified athletic trainers for their time and personal true stories for a health care profession where new experiences are never ending. Keith would also like to thank his wonderful family (Betsy, Erin, and Tyler), for their continued support through all of the years of clinical and educational athletic training.

Francis Feld would like to thank the athletic trainers that were willing to contribute to this text. We can learn from history, but all too often these episodes are lost to time because they were not told. Confucius said, "Study the past if you would define the future," and it is our hope that the next generation of athletic trainers benefit from these experiences. Francis would also like to thank his wife Christine for her love and support.

Robert O. Blanc would like to thank all of the athletic trainers whose stories have, and will, pass on to future generations what this profession is truly about. The professionalism, caring, and dedication that is shown in the details of these stories and the millions of untold stories make what we do so special. Robert would also like to thank his wife Peggy for her unmatched love and support.

Contributing Authors

Adam Annaccone, EdD, ATC, CES, PES (True Story #30)
Baylor Scott & White Sports Therapy & Research

Morgan Cooper Bagley, PhD, AT, ATC (True Story #16)
University of Mount Union

Robert O. Blanc, MS, LAT, ATC, EMT-P (True Story #9)
University of Pittsburgh

Richard Burr, MS, LAT, ATC, CSCS (True Story #31)
Babson College

Paul A. Cacolice, PhD, LAT, ATC, CSCS (True Story #29)
Westfield State University

Douglas Casa, PhD, ATC, FNAK, FACSM, FNATA (True Story #4)
University of Connecticut

Robert J. Casmus, MS, ATC (True Story #18)
Catawba College

James Cerullo, PhD, ATC, CSCS (True Story #10)
State University of New York—Oneonta

Kevin Conley, PhD, LAT, ATC (True Story #6)
University of Pittsburgh

Larry Cooper, MS, LAT, ATC (True Stories #3 and #25)
Penn Trafford High School

Bill Couts, LAT, ATC (True Story #33)
University of Pittsburgh Medical Center Sports Medicine

Tim Dunlavey, MS, LAT, ATC (True Story #22)
PGA Golf Tour

Francis Feld, DNP, CRNA, LAT, ATC, NRP (True Story #20)
University of Pittsburgh Medical Center Passavant Hospital

Tim Giel, MS, LAT, ATC (True Story #23)
Avonworth High School

Keith M. Gorse, EdD, LAT, ATC (True Story #32)
Duquesne University

Al Green, MEd, LAT, ATC, EMT (True Story #34)
Florida Southern College

Michael Hanley, ATC, LAT (True Story #13)
East Carolina University

Timothy J. Henry, PhD, ATC (True Story #24)
State University of New York—Brockport

Valerie Herzog, EdD, LAT, ATC (True Story #5)
Weber State University

Peggy A. Houglum, PhD (True Story #11)
Duquesne University (retired)

Ryan Johnson, LAT, ATC (True Story #17)
Avonworth High School

Kyle Johnston, MS, ATC, LAT (True Story #19)
University of Louisville

Blake LeBlanc, PT, DPT, ATC, LAT (True Story #19)
University of Louisville

Sarah Manspeaker, PhD, LAT, ATC (True Story #15)
Duquesne University

Kate McCartney, MS, LAT, ATC (True Story #1)
University of Pittsburgh

Ryan McGovern, MS, LAT, ATC (True Story #21)
Duquesne University

Randy McGuire, MS, ATC, LAT (True Story #28)
Georgetown College

David H. Perrin, PhD, ATC, FNATA (True Story #2)
University of Utah

Marirose Radelet, MS, PT, LAT, ATC (True Stories #7 and #8)
Northshore Stallions Midget Football League

Richard Ray, EdD, ATC (True Story #35)
Hope College

Gaetano Sanchioli, MS, LAT, ATC, PES (True Story #27)
University of Pittsburgh Medical Center and Carrick High School

Jeff Shields, MEd, LAT, ATC, CEAS (True Story #14)
Central PA Rehabilitation Services, Inc Physical Therapy

Rebecca L. Stearns, PhD, ATC (True Story #4)
University of Connecticut

Giampietro L. Vairo, PhD, LAT, ATC (True Story #26)
Penn State University

Sam Zuege, MS, ATC, LAT (True Story #19)
University of Louisville

Mary Mundrane-Zweiacher, PT, ATC, CHT (True Story #12)
Bayhealth Medical Center

PREFACE

True Stories From the Athletic Training Room is intended to give the reader insight into the athletic training profession with real-life stories that may occur in each of the 5 domains of athletic training education. It is the intent of this textbook to provide the reader with many true-to-life stories that have occurred and been shared by certified athletic trainers who are currently working with industrial, high schools, colleges, professional teams, and sports medicine clinics. It is our intent to include true stories listed for each of the domains listed in the National Athletic Trainers' Association Board of Certification.

After a few years of building on this idea, it is pleasing to see our concept take shape and to see this textbook become a reality. It is our hope that *True Stories From the Athletic Training Room* will be an asset to the student athletic trainer, the certified athletic trainer, and any other health care provider, and that it will serve as a promotional tool for the athletic training profession.

Domain I

Injury and Illness Prevention
and Wellness Protection

KLIPPEL-TRENAUNAY SYNDROME IN COLLEGIATE VOLLEYBALL

Kate McCartney, MS, LAT, ATC

KEY TERMS

Klippel-Trenaunay Syndrome | General Medical Disorders

In my very first year working women's volleyball at the Division I collegiate level, I had an incoming freshman athlete with Klippel-Trenaunay syndrome. Not only was it important for me in my career to learn the ins and outs of the game of volleyball, I also had to learn about a very rare disease that had very little information available and lacked research on the effects of participating in athletics with such a disease. I was working with a specialist that was extremely difficult to get in contact with and failed to understand of the game and my role as an athletic trainer. I also had to help guide the athlete through some very difficult decision making. This situation taught me about who I am as an athletic trainer more than any other situation that I have been faced with.

TRUE STORY #1

The athlete did not alert us to any medical conditions in her preseason paperwork despite the request for a full medical history, nor did she bring anything to the attention of our team physicians at the time of physicals so when her first symptoms arose I was very unaware of what I would be dealing with.

When the symptoms first presented, the athlete came to me with distinct bumps across her left forearm, and extreme pain, especially upon palpation. I scheduled her an appointment with our team physician for 2 days later and decided to hold her from all activity until she could see him.

Before the athlete could see our team physicians, her parents scheduled a meeting with me and the coaching staff to bring to light that the athlete was very recently diagnosed with "a very mild case" of Klippel-Trenaunay syndrome. They explained

Gorse KM, Feld F, Blanc RO, eds.
True Stories From the Athletic Training Room (pp 3-30).
© 2018 SLACK Incorporated.

that it was "what Casey Martin, the golfer, had," and that "this thing in her arm happens very rarely." Her parents then took her to the specialist that they had in New York that treats the very rare disease while my team physician and myself took it upon ourselves to now learn everything we could about the disease.

Klippel-Trenaunay syndrome is a birth defect that prevents proper formation of the blood and lymph vessels. It usually effects one quarter of the body and can result on local gigantism of shrinkage. It also greatly increases the risk of blood clot development and, therefore, pulmonary embolism as well as heart disease. In Casey Martin's case, it affected his right leg and was the reason he was granted permission to use a golf cart on the Professional Golfers' Association Tour. In this athlete's case, however, the effected body part was her left arm. As a Division I setter, the use of that arm was extremely important. Our team physician decided that, we as a medical staff, would yield to the specialist in New York as he is one of the few that treats the disease and take his recommendations on her return to play.

In New York, the athlete underwent a two-fold procedure. First, debulking was performed and the masses that had developed in her arm were removed. Next, the specialist went through and cauterized the vessels that led to the locations of where the formations had been with the intention of preventing further development. The athlete returned with paperwork from the specialist requesting the student be out for one week before gradually returning to activity.

After a week, we very slowly worked the athlete back into volleyball. Initially, we just working on getting her back into shape and being mindful about the amount the athlete used her left arm. Before she could return to full practices, the bumps returned. We promptly pulled her and attempted to reach her specialist in New York. We were unable at this point to speak with him directly, but decided it was best that she return to his office to follow up.

When she returned to New York, she underwent another procedure. It was the same but on a slightly smaller scale. The specialist admitted that maybe he had been too aggressive and recommended sitting out 2 full weeks with a much slower return to play. This same cycle repeated itself 2 more times over the next couple of months. As soon as the athlete would attempt to return to play, even at a light to moderate level, the symptoms would present gain. We modified her activity by removing her from all extra cardio and weight lifting in an attempt to get her back to playing volleyball. Unfortunately, none of our modifications were successful. With each of the 3 subsequent procedures, I attempted to contact the specialist, but was unable to reach him. My team physician also tried multiple times to communicate with him, but to no avail.

Now 3 months and 3 surgeries into her volleyball career, we decided that the athlete should sit out the remainder of the semester to hopefully allow for an ample amount of time to heal. We would redshirt her so that she wouldn't lose any eligibility and we would ensure her that she could get properly conditioned back to volleyball at a very gradual pace. It was late October at this point and we decided we wouldn't worry about getting her back into volleyball until the following August.

At this point, the athlete was not coming to workouts with the team as she had decided to redshirt, so I had little contact with her other than checking in periodically to see how she was healing and what activity she was doing at the time. Without our knowledge, the athlete returned to her club volleyball gym where she continued to work out and over the course of the next 5 months, underwent 2 more surgeries, totaling 6 in approximately 8 months' time. It was at this point that the specialist finally contacted our team physician, bringing to our attention that more procedures had occurred and to discuss what we had been doing with the athlete.

Our team physician put the specialist in touch with me. When I first spoke with him he was very accusatory, questioning the level of activity that I must be putting on his patient. I explained our current situation, which he understood, though he was adamant that volleyball couldn't be enough to exasperate the symptoms and that there must be something else we were doing with her that led to the increase in symptoms. He also explained to me that at this point if she continued her current rate of surgeries, she would lose her arm completely before the age of 25 because she would lose so many blood vessels. He felt at this point that she could continue to play volleyball so long as she refrained from everything else.

Another meeting was scheduled with the athlete, her parents, the coaching staff and myself. The coaches and I expressed our concerns, referencing the risks that I had recently learned of. We recommended that she discontinue her volleyball career at this point, but that we would allow her to continue so long as she was fully honest with us and only worked out under our supervision and recommendation. The mother seemed receptive to the idea, but her father was adamant that she continue. As a family, they decided to continue.

Over the summer months, we did very little with the athlete and she responded well, but as we started back with some volleyball we found ourselves in the same situation. Another surgery was scheduled and again another big conversation about what to do next. It occurred to me at this point that the specialist maybe didn't understand the demand that volleyball placed on the body. I too had just learned that this version of volleyball was very different from the gym class game that I remembered, so I sent him some videos of Division I women's volleyball and he was extremely surprised at the level of impact and activity. For the first time the specialist admitted that maybe it wasn't in her best interest to continue; however, he would continue to perform the surgeries as necessary if that's what his patient wanted.

Now after talking again with the athlete's specialist and all of us, the athlete's mother was fully on board with discontinuing her volleyball career. The father on the other hand was not, demanding that they get another opinion and that it was our fault that she continued to become symptomatic. The athlete was then placed in a very tough position as her father had been her life-long coach and though it was ultimately her decision she was afraid to let her father down. I tried to remain supportive of her as she weighed both sides. I educated her as much as I could on the risks, and I recommended she seek some outside counseling and take her time in making the decision when she was ready.

Before the start of the next school year the athlete did make the decision to discontinue her volleyball career. Even though it was a very difficult decision, it was the right one for her. At this point, since she wouldn't be playing, she decided to transfer to a different school farther from home where she could hopefully let the game of volleyball go all together. Now at the age of 24 she has only had to undergo 2 more surgeries and has the promise of a much healthier future.

REFLECTION

The biggest take away I had as an athletic trainer dealing with this case, first and foremost, was the importance of developing a trusting relationship with student athletes and parents. Originally, the family tried to hide the disease because they feared that their daughter would not receive a scholarship or that we would take that scholarship away from her. Secondly, making sure everyone that is included in the team of care should be on the same page and aware of what the expectations of the patient will be. Lastly, it is important to take a step back from the athletic realm to make the right decision. As an athletic trainer, my goal has always been to find a way to get an athlete back into play, no matter what. This was my first instance where playing volleyball was detrimental to the health and well-being of the student athlete, so helping her to realize that in her own time became my primary goal. There were some strong emotions and resistance, but I learned that it isn't important for everyone to like you. In the end, it is important to reach the best decision for the student athlete.

TAKING A STAND FOR THE HEALTH AND SAFETY OF ATHLETES

David H. Perrin, PhD, ATC, FNATA

KEY TERMS

Injury Prevention | Conflict Resolution

Athletic trainers sometimes find themselves in difficult situations where he or she must take a stand against the coaches with whom they work in support of the health and safety of the athletes under his or her care. Examples include removing athletes from dangerous environmental exposure (eg, lightening, excessive heat or humidity) and resisting pressure to prematurely return athletes to competition following injury (eg, concussion). The difficulty of these situations can be exacerbated when the athletic trainer is young and inexperienced or lacks support from his or her supervisor. This is the story of an athletic trainer's first week in his first job out of graduate school, just weeks after becoming certified. The scene is a major Division I university athletic program and an athletic training room for which the young athletic trainer had administrative responsibility (while reporting to a head athletic trainer in another facility). One of the sports practiced in this athletic training facility was wrestling, led by a long-time coach with a rather domineering personality. Upon reporting to work, the athletic trainer encountered a rather unique device in the athletic training room, designed to facilitate dehydration and weight loss among collegiate wrestlers.

TRUE STORY #2

This athletic trainer's first position was at a major Division I university where he was responsible for the administration of one of 3 athletic training rooms. The athletic training facility provided health care to several men's sports, including soccer, basketball, wrestling, cross country, track and field, and baseball. The facility was equipped with most of the standard equipment found in athletic training rooms in the late 1970s, including taping and treatment tables, ice machine, therapeutic modalities, and an assortment of therapeutic exercise equipment. There was, however, one exception.

Located in the middle of the athletic training room was a white box that looked like an old-fashioned washing machine. The box had a hole in the top, and inside the box were several dozen light bulbs. The intercollegiate wrestlers sat in the box with only their head visible through the hole in the top. The light bulbs were switched on to generate significant heat within the box for the purpose of inducing sweat and weight loss. This was, of course, a strategy to aid the wrestlers in "making weight" prior to wrestling matches. The athletic trainer expressed his concern over the presence of the device to the head athletic trainer.

The athletic trainer was faced with several options. One was to accept the presence of this device as a part of the *status quo* and as an acceptable "modality" to induce weight loss in wrestlers. Another was for the athletic trainer to discuss his concerns with the wrestling coach. Among the concerns regarding this machine were the unhealthy and potentially dangerous effects of this device on the wrestlers, the professional liability for the athletic trainer with the device being in the athletic training room, and the negative impact the device had on the professional environment of this health care facility. The athletic trainer chose to express his concerns to the wrestling coach, and to take a stand that the existence of the device was unacceptable, not only in the athletic training room, but anywhere that would make it accessible to the wrestlers.

The initial response of the wrestling coach was far from understanding. He felt that this young, relatively inexperienced athletic trainer was in no way going to dictate how he conducted his wrestling program. His position was that the box had been effective in helping wrestlers make weight and that he had never encountered any problems with its use. The athletic trainer reiterated his position that the device would have to go.

At an impasse, the athletic trainer again expressed his concern to the head athletic trainer. The wrestling coach conveyed his position to the athletic director, who was somewhat equivocal on the matter. The head athletic trainer (and probably medical director) stood with the athletic trainer. After some time, the box was removed from the athletic training room and dismantled. The wrestling coach was quite unhappy and for some time the relationship between the coach and athletic trainer was strained. Over time, however, the relationship between the coach and athletic trainer became quite collegial and even friendly.

REFLECTION

While one's first position as a certified athletic trainer is exciting, it can also be daunting and overwhelming. The challenges one faces can be exacerbated by relationships with new colleagues who have long histories and deeply embedded cultures within the work place. The following guidelines may be useful in helping to address and resolve difficult situations:

- The health and safety of the athletes under your care must always be your primary concern.

- Attempt to resolve potential conflicts by having a conversation in person, not via email, with the person with whom you have the issue.

- Ensure you have the support of your supervisor before taking a stand that might threaten the stability of your job.

- If unsuccessful in rectifying a situation that does not meet the standards of best practices in athletic training, document your position in writing with your supervisor.

- Decide if the work setting is appropriate for you or if it unacceptably comprises your morals and principles.

The aforementioned scenario occurred 40 years ago. Thankfully, many advances have been made in the manner by which athletic trainers provide health care to athletes. Challenges still remain, for example, a recent article in *The Chronicle of Higher Education* addressed the challenges athletic trainers face in providing proper care to athletes receiving concussion. An alarming number of athletic trainers face threats to their jobs when taking a stand against coaches relative to the premature return of athletes to competition. Athletic trainers must remain diligent in ensuring that the health and safety of athletes under their care is foremost in their minds without threat of compromise.

An Unknown Visitor

Larry Cooper, MS, LAT, ATC

KEY TERMS

Emergency Action Plan | Documentation | Networking

The motto of most teachers is, "get to know students." The same applies for athletic trainers but we usually take it one step further and prepare for anything because anything can happen at any time. I get to know many students and those that are athletes even better. Sometimes you spend as much time with them as you do with your own children. I try to develop relationships that will continue way past graduation. When you are in a school or community for a long period, you also have the benefit of getting to know families and that might include aunts, uncles, and grandparents. It is something that I have come to enjoy in my nearly 3 decades of service to my community.

True Story #3

It was the time of year that I enjoy the most, Christmas break, when alumni often return to tell us about their college experience, visit with former teammates and coaches or to practice with a team so that they can maintain their level of conditioning. It was very cold that morning and I prepared for practices (wrestling, basketball and swimming/diving) like I always did. I made my rounds talking with the coaches and had returned to the athletic training room to supervise the rehabilitation of a few athletes. It was a typical day, low key, relaxed and quiet, something that I have enjoyed over the Christmas holiday break for years. Suddenly, there was a yell for my name from a girls' basketball player. The tone and decibel level heightened my awareness immediately. She said, "come quick, there is someone down in the front hallway." I grabbed my pack and took off running.

I asked her questions. She had no idea who it was that was injured but did say that he was shaking, unconscious, and there was blood everywhere. It took me about 20 to 25 seconds to reach the area and yes, there was blood everywhere. It was dark in the hallway because it was over holiday break, and custodial and maintenance staff had off. Close examination showed it was a former student athlete of our school and he was starting to regain consciousness. My instinct was to stabilize the head since we didn't know his injury mechanism, but he was unconsciousness and there was blood.

At this time, my fellow athletic trainer appeared and started to go through a full neurological examination. Fortunately, there were no deficits. Discussion with the injured athlete revealed that he did not recall anything. The last thing that he recalled was walking down the hallway. Piecing bits and pieces of the puzzle together, we concluded that he had had a seizure episode, fell, hit his head on the hard tile floor and that was when we found him. Fortunately, I knew his parents' phone number from previous injuries to him and his siblings. I called them immediately and discussed what had happened as they drove to the school.

When you live in a small community there are stories that fly around, some factual, some half-truths, some just plain lies. I had heard that this young man had a seizure over the summer but they attributed it to playing a version of a *Call of Duty* (Activision) video game. When his father came to get him, I suggested that, considering what happened today and what had happened over the summer, he get a full neurological evaluation. While we were talking, he called his primary care physician and he stated the same thing. The father did take him to the local emergency room for X-rays and computerized tomography scan which were negative. The follow up appointment with his neurologist was not so kind. He was diagnosed with epilepsy and was unable to drive or return to his sport for that year. It took a while for his medication to get to the point where he could function without issues; however, this athlete could return to his sport of choice and all activities within 9 months.

REFLECTION

This situation could have had a much different outcome if we had not known the athlete or if the girls' basketball player had not walked down that hallway to the locker room. Fortunately, everything resolved with only minor issues for the athlete. It did however change the way that the athletic department handled practices and visitors. Whenever there is a serious injury, we take the time to review our steps, the care given, and try to evaluate it so that we improve. This was no exception. No longer are alumni or visitors allowed to attend or participate in practices or conditioning sessions. This is something that was enforced across the board with all sports at all levels. Now all sports are following state athletic association bylaws. There also seems to be more communication between the athletic training staff about practice schedules over the holidays and coaches seem to have a better understanding and appreciation for the job that we perform on a daily basis. One thing is for sure, alumni and visitors are never permitted to join our practices. We do not know their current health status and do not have contact information readily available. This puts those athletes, the school district, and the athletic trainers in a very litigious situation.

RETURNING A COMPLICATED EXERTIONAL HEAT STROKE CASE TO ACTIVITY

Rebecca L. Stearns, PhD, ATC and
Douglas Casa, PhD, ATC, FNAK, FACSM, FNATA

KEY TERMS

Exertional Heat Stroke | Heat Illness | Heat Tolerance Test

On August 12, 2013, Gavin Class, then 21 years old, 6 feet, 4 inches, and 300 pounds, was preparing for his upcoming football season at Towson University. During a conditioning session, Gavin collapsed, lost consciousness and was assumed to be suffering from exertional heat stroke (EHS). Gavin was placed into a cold water immersion tub. Simultaneously, emergency medical services was called and arrived within 5 minutes into cooling. Gavin was removed for transport to the local emergency department; however, his body temperature was not assessed until admission to the hospital where his temperature was still 108°F.

Gavin's hospital cooling treatment consisted of ice bags placed over his body. At this point Gavin approached the dangerous 30 minute mark, where complications and potentially death from EHS drastically increases when body temperature is not sufficiently lowered to under 104°F. Without aggressive cooling, his body began to feel the complications of EHS. He slipped into a coma, and in the ensuing 6 weeks he spent at the hospital he had a total of 14 surgeries which included and addressed a liver transplant, pancreatitis, pneumonia, appendicitis, shingles, and a collapsed lung. Miraculously, he did survive. Given the inappropriate care, Gavin was lucky to be alive. Still, this was only the first step in his recovery.

TRUE STORY #4

The Recovery Process

Recovery from EHS can be a relatively uncomplicated process when immediate and aggressive cooling is completed within 30 minutes of the onset of the EHS (and body temperature is lowered to under 104°F). However, when treatment is delayed, recovery becomes complicated and typically requires additional consultation and expert advice. For Gavin's case, Gavin and the university's athletic trainers sought the advice of the Korey Stringer Institute (KSI). In August of 2014, a full year after his EHS, Gavin came to KSI to have a heat tolerance test (HTT) performed.

The HTT was developed by the Israeli army and has been adopted and used within the US military as a guiding tool in complicated cases of EHS. While no other exertional test exists to assess the body's ability to tolerate exercise heat stress, it has also come into use within the athletic setting for specialized cases. The test itself consists of walking for 2 hours in a hot environment (104°F, 40% humidity) at a 2% incline at 3.1 mph. Passing criteria consists of a rectal temperature remaining below 38.5°C (101.3°F) with demonstration of a plateau in rectal temperature in the last hour. Other supporting information is also collected such as a heart rate that remains below 150 bpm. While this test has its own limitations, it has been found to be a good tool to guide and assist in determining an individual's baseline ability to tolerate low intensity exercise in the heat.

Gavin failed his first HTT in August of 2014, though it was not with finality that these results were delivered. Upon looking at Gavin's case, it was determined that Gavin had many modifiable factors that could be addressed to help improve his heat tolerance; fitness, above all being a main focus. Gavin was provided instructions on how he could improve these modifiable factors and 5 months to improve before coming back for a re-evaluation in February of 2015. This time he passed the test.

While passing the HTT was another step in his recovery, it did not guarantee that any future risk was completely absent; however, failing a HTT gives a clear indication that intense exercise in the heat is not prudent at that time. Even in healthy athletes there is always a risk of exertional heat illness. Even so, there are many examples of successful return to activity cases from EHS within both sport and military. For this reason, the following recommendations were provided to the Towson medical team to help guide Gavin's continued recovery and progression back to full participation:

1. Perform a progression of low to high intensity exercise in cool environments over the course of weeks and months.

2. Following #1 above, the introduction of workouts performed in the heat should gradually work up in duration and frequency over the course of 2 to 4 weeks, adhering to a specific heat acclimatization program. This is standard policy for any introduction of athletes to exercise in the heat.

3. We suggest monitoring body temperature (specifically with an ingestible thermistor) when performing new and unique exercise or conditioning sessions, especially when done in warm to hot environments. This may represent a total of 3 to 4 weeks of the year (ie the first 1 to 2 weeks of spring football and the first 1 to 2 weeks of preseason in August), as these are generally the riskiest times of the year for heat illness. Monitoring would help to guarantee that participation is safe and confirm that there is no need for exercise modification. Utilizing an ingestible thermistor is relatively cost effective, quick to assemble and reliable, which makes it ideal for these scenarios. As a second level of security, a rectal thermometer should be on hand if a confirmatory measure needs to be made.

4. It is important to continue to monitor fluid needs, as fluid needs will increase with warm weather exposure and an increase in your fitness (or the opposite with declines in either of these). Mitigating fluid losses to avoid reductions of greater than 2% will be a great tool to help regulate temperature during exercise.

5. All exercise progression should be done at the discretion and under direct observation of a medical professional. It is always important to monitor athletes for signs and symptoms of illness and modify practices based on extreme weather conditions.

Return-to-Play Decisions

While KSI's involvement past this point was limited, KSI cleared Gavin to begin a return-to-play progression with the suggestion that his body temperature be monitored during his initial return to football (at a minimum). As of April 2015, however, Gavin was not allowed to return to practice since his team physician refused to clear him for football. Her main reason was cited as the inability to ensure he would not have another EHS. The university stated that it could not manage his risk for EHS "with any reasonable restriction or accommodation." This was in reference to the recommendation that Gavin take an ingestible thermometer during preseason and have it periodically measure by the athletic training staff. This accommodation would cost $30 to $40 per ingestible thermometer as well as a few hundred dollars to lease the receiver to read the body temperature, all of which the family offered to pay for. This inability to accommodate Gavin's rehabilitation also stemmed from the team physician's belief that the athletic trainers were not qualified to monitor body temperature, nor did the physician feel that athletic trainers were true medical professionals.

Unfortunately, Gavin's team physician never consulted with KSI regarding her decision. We believe that, given the opportunity, we could have at a minimum agreed upon and provided a potential path forward for Gavin's rehabilitation, which would have provided an opportunity to assess his readiness to return.

Following these decisions, the family brought a lawsuit against the university. The U.S. District Court, led by Judge Richard D. Bennett who was very critical of Towson's arguments for not allowing Gavin to return to play, cleared Class to play. From our understanding, this is the first case in the country where a federal judge has ordered a university to allow an athlete to play against the decision of the university. This is also the first case where a judge has ruled that heatstroke is a disability. While all of this was positive momentum for Gavin, the university quickly repealed the ruling, which sent the case to the U.S. Court of Appeals in Richmond, Virginia.

Prior to the appeals court date and, in order to provide additional support and documentation of Gavin's recovery, in June of 2015 (2 years after his EHS) Gavin came to KSI again to have additional testing done. This time, the heat test was performed at a greater intensity and, in a way, that was designed to mimic, as best as possible, the common demands placed on National Collegiate Athletic Association (NCAA) linemen like Gavin. Based on normative data for high intensity exercise experienced during preseason, NCAA linemen complete about 1.6 miles at 60% of their VO2 max (with usual breaks that occur during a normal preseason practice). If performed continuously on a treadmill at this speed/intensity, Gavin could attain this value within 19 minutes.

The test was again performed in the same environmental conditions as his previous HTT (104°F and 40% humidity). During the test Gavin went so far as to complete 50 minutes of exercise at 60% of his VO2 max while staying under a safe and expected rectal temperature (103°F). This equated to completing 265% of the estimated workload necessary for preseason practices in extreme heat. KSI concluded that by being more fit, more acclimatized, and consuming appropriate amounts of fluids likely aided in a successful test. The testing environment was also beyond any environment we would expect exercise sessions to be held. This would logically allow these results to be applied to practice sessions in any environmental conditions less than or equal to these, per NCAA guidelines. This gave us an even greater demonstration of Gavin's road to recovery and ability to handle expected workloads in extreme heat.

At this point we suggested the following to Gavin:

1. Continue to participate fully in summer conditioning workouts and fully participate with regularly scheduled football practices.

2. Continue to perform conditioning workouts outside in order to maintain heat acclimatization status.

3. Continue to follow the mandated NCAA heat acclimatization guidelines for any introduction of equipment, as these will help slowly introduce and progress you to the next and last progression step for return-to-play, which is exercise in the heat with protective equipment.

4. Monitor your body temperature (via ingestible thermistors with rectal temperature as a backup) when performing new and unique exercise or conditioning sessions, especially when done in warm to hot environments. This may represent a total of 3 to 4 weeks of the year (ie the first 1 to 2 weeks of spring football and the first 1 to 2 weeks of preseason in August when new exercise sessions or equipment is introduced.), as these are generally the riskiest times of the year for heat illness. Monitoring would help to guarantee our participation is safe and confirm that there is no need for exercise modification.

5. Monitor your fluid needs and match your fluid losses so as to consume equal to or greater than 50% to 60% of your expected losses but not to exceed 90% to 100% of your needs. Fluid needs will increase with warm weather exposure and with increases in your fitness.

6. All exercise progression should be done at the discretion and under direct observation of a medical professional. It is always important to monitor athletes for signs and symptoms of illness, have emergency treatment protocols and equipment ready, and modify practices based on extreme weather conditions.

Lastly, Gavin returned to court to hear the final verdict. It was at the Court of Appeals that Judge Paul V. Niemeyer ruled that Towson appropriately followed its policy regarding the return-to-play of injured athletes. He wrote, "Giving deference to Towson University's judgment, as we are required to do, we uphold its determination..." This ultimately ended all hopes that Gavin would be able to play his senior year at Towson University.

While Gavin was unable to complete this senior year at Towson, his athletic career has not stopped. Gavin decided to direct his work toward the Donate Life Transplant Games, which he competed in June of 2016. It is a multisport festival event produced by the Transplant Games of America for individuals who have undergone life-saving transplant surgeries (competition events are open to living donors and transplant recipients). Gavin earned 5 medals in 3 sports, 2 in swimming, 2 in track and one in racquetball. He hopes to train for the 2017 World Transplant Games in Málaga, Spain.

Our hope by sharing this story with you is to remind medical providers that immediate, aggressive whole body immersion within 10 minutes of collapse has resulted not only in 100% survival from EHS, but rather when this life saving modality is not applied, we see deaths or lingering complications as in this and other cases. Without immediate cold water immersion applied for an effective duration, the path to recovery becomes complicated and requires specialized assessment for lingering complications, in which also places future potential for healthy, safe and full sport participation at risk.

REFLECTION

As a final note, we would like to make it clear that the authors believe that team physicians should have authority to determine the course of an athlete's medical care, independent of pressures that could be exerted from a direction unrelated to health and safety (ie the desire for a star player to play in a critical game). We also believe, however, that in the course of a specialized and complicated medical condition, such as Gavin's, additional medical insight should be discussed and sought from those that specialize in that area. While KSI has consulted with, tested and treated hundreds of EHS cases, this was the university physician's first EHS case. While KSI suggested a graduated return to play, it was not intended to allow full return to participation without certain steps and precautions in place. Certainly, as with any serious injury, a progression would be expected, but at the end of which a final determination of playing ability could be made. The authors feel that Gavin was not provided the opportunity to progress through these steps. The authors believe the accommodations and restrictions were absolutely reasonable within the realm of a practicing athletic trainer at a Division I football program and have also been successfully implemented at many levels of sport within football (the closest example being Hunter Knighton from Miami University). The authors would like to emphasize that the need for specialized care can also be mitigated by ensuring that a rectal temperature of 104°F or lower has been confirmed prior to emergency medical services transport and removal from the life-saving cold water immersion treatment. Not only has this been demonstrated to be effective at saving victims of EHS, but also in avoiding complicated outcomes such as this case.

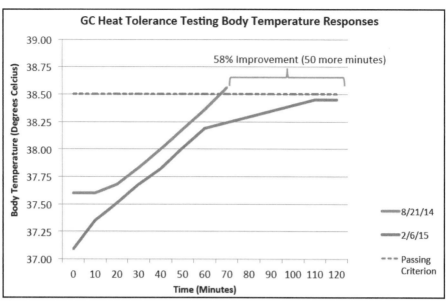

Figure 4-1. Heat tolerance test graph.

Conference Planning Saves Lives

Valerie Herzog, EdD, LAT, ATC

Key Terms

Conference Planning | Exertional Heat Stroke | Continuing Education

---

Getting involved in serving the athletic training profession can have many benefits. You may build your skill set, expand your network, find a great job, or just feel a sense of satisfaction from the act of service. Sometimes though, it can pay off in ways that you might never have imagined.

True Story #5

When I moved to Utah in 2004, it was the first time that I had lived west of the Mississippi. I didn't know anyone in the state or even in the region. I was excited to get to know other athletic trainers in the area and build a new professional community. I thought that speaking at a conference would be a good way to start meeting people and getting involved, but I wasn't sure where to start.

I looked on the Rocky Mountain Athletic Trainers' Association (RMATA) website for information about their annual conference. I couldn't find any information regarding how to submit a presentation proposal, but I did find the contact information for the individual who was in charge of planning the program. I sent him an email to express my interest in presenting and some topics that I would be comfortable presenting. He responded to let me know that he was stepping down as the committee chair and that they would need some new committee members. The new committee would then select the speakers for the conference, so he encouraged me to consider joining the committee.

I emailed Lisa Walker, the current President of the RMATA, to ask her how to apply for the conference committee. She asked me to send in a letter of interest and resume, which I did, and then I waited. A few weeks later, she contacted me to let me know that I had been approved to join the conference committee and that they would like me to chair the committee.

I was very unsure about this and explained to Lisa that I had never been involved with conference planning before. I also had never attended the RMATA conference so I had no idea what it was like. She told me that Dr. Ken Knight had assured her that I would do a great job. This also surprised me as I had only briefly met Dr. Knight once or twice in the previous 2 years. Lisa further explained that it wouldn't be too difficult because the conference was going to be in Salt Lake City, near Ogden, where I was living. I just needed to fill the 3-day program with local speakers. Again, I explained that I just moved to Utah and didn't really know anyone, but she assured me that I would figure it out. I was more than a little nervous about this enormous task, but was excited to have been presented with the opportunity, so I agreed to do it.

I started making calls to anyone I had met in Utah and found everyone to be extremely helpful in identifying potential speakers. One of the speakers we brought in that year was Dr. Doug Casa. He had contacted me with a desire to speak on the management of exertional heat stroke. My speaker budget was limited, but Gatorade (PepsiCo) was going to pay for his travel so we added him to the program. I was thrilled to be filling the program with interesting topics and a slate of impressive speakers. Despite some logistical issues (such as forgetting to print copies of the program or creating speaker evaluations in advance) the conference team helped me figure it out and assured me that it was actually a pretty good conference.

One of the most interesting presentations at the conference was Dr. Casa's recommendations on managing exertional heat stroke. He introduced the idea that we should be monitoring core body temperature with a rectal thermometer and submerging the athlete in a bath of ice water prior to transporting them to the hospital for more advanced care. This treatment protocol was a significant change from what most of us had learned and created a great deal of discussion in the hallways. It was hard to ignore that when this had been done in the military, not a single death had occurred.

Jeff Speckman was a local athletic trainer who attended the RMATA conference in April of 2006 and listened to Dr. Casa's presentation. He immediately took the information back to his physician group as they were already getting ready for the Ogden marathon that June. Jeff Speckman was insistent that they implement the new recommendations, but it wasn't easy to make such large changes in such a short amount of time. The athletic trainers and physicians worked together over the next 6 weeks to make it happen, and it paid off.

Jeff Speckman was the athletic trainer in the medical tent with a medical team including physicians. A 35-year-old male runner collapsed at the finish line of the marathon. He was initially unresponsive, pale, and clammy. His rectal temperature was 41.7°C (107°F). He was immediately transferred to an ice-water pool where his clothes were stripped and he had ice placed to his groin, axilla, femoral arteries, and neck. He was given supplemental oxygen, 2 IVs were placed, and a saline infusion was started (running through ice water). After 30 minutes, his temperature dropped to 39°C (102°F). He was then transported to a local hospital.

The runner was treated in the hospital and by physicians for the next few days as he still had some lingering blood chemistry issues, but he was able to make a full recovery. His life was saved by the work of the medical team and through the implementation of the new treatment protocols that had been presented at the RMATA conference. The runner and the medical team returned to the RMATA conference in 2009 to tell this story and encourage others to implement this protocol as well if they had not already done so.

Many small steps were taken that saved a life that day. I feel that my step to agree to plan the conference was the smallest contribution, but it triggered a change in procedure. Dr. Casa was brave enough to push for a radical new treatment protocol and delivered a compelling presentation. Jeff Speckman was energized to action and was able to convince the marathon's medical team to change their treatment plans in a very short period of time. The medical team then saved a life and paid it forward by sharing their success at the same conference where the story began.

REFLECTION

This story is about several athletic trainers who all stepped up in different ways to serve the profession. A team of health care professionals also worked together to implement new accepted practices based on quality evidence. The ultimate result was that a life was saved. The runner even paid it forward by sharing his story with the health care team to continue educating others. This is what it's all about. This is why we go to work every day. Athletic trainers make a difference every day in the lives of our athletes and patients, sometimes, we even save their lives.

NEWLY CERTIFIED FOOTBALL OUTCOME

Kevin Conley, PhD, LAT, ATC

KEY TERMS

Trauma | Triage | Hypovolemic Shock | Stabilization

As a newly certified athletic trainer working on my own for the first time at a small high school, I was confronted with a situation on the football field where the outcome was merely a source of embarrassment for me, but which could have proven more dire for the injured student athlete.

TRUE STORY #6

On an early fall Saturday morning, I was preparing to cover a high school football game, only the fourth time I had done so on my own as a recently certified athletic trainer. The pregame rituals were always the same. I arrived 2 hours before kickoff to prepare the players and set up the field. I also had to meet with the local emergency medical services (EMS) personnel who would be on site to cover the game in the event of a serious trauma requiring more advanced care or transportation. On this particular Saturday, a seasoned emergency medical technician was accompanied by a junior partner, neither of whom had ever gone on to a playing field to assist an injured patient. As game time approached, I felt prepared and confident that a solid plan was in place in the event of a significant injury and everyone involved knew their respective roles.

Midway through the second quarter, a senior wide receiver jumped, arms outstretched, to catch a pass from the quarterback. When he landed with the ball, he was struck from his right side by an opposing player attempting to make a tackle. The crown of the defender's helmet struck the receiver's right arm above the elbow, pinning it to his side as they both fell to the ground. Once the tackler got off the pile, I quickly realized that my athlete was not getting up. Instead, he was laying on his back holding his right arm.

As I approached the injured player, I saw he was very calm. When I asked him what had happened, he informed me, in no uncertain terms, that he broke his arm. Wanting to confirm this myself, I grasped his upper arm and immediately felt the sensation of crepitus. This could only mean one thing; this young man had a complete fracture of his humerus.

An immediate adrenalin rush came over me as I took a brief moment to recognize that this was the most serious injury I had encountered at this point in my fledgling career. After quickly collecting my thoughts, I confirmed that the athlete had indeed broken his arm, but that he was in good hands and I was going to see to it that his arm was well taken care of. I asked him a few questions to ascertain his level of alertness and again was struck by the degree of clam he was exhibiting. One of the coaches had come onto the field at this point and I explained my finding. He immediately suggested we have the ambulance come over and take the player off the field.

I knew that this was probably the most prudent course of action, but still, my instincts told me that I could handle the situation and get this athlete off the field on my own without the need to rely on others to assist me. Not sensing anything that would keep the athlete from standing up, I instructed the coach to go to the athlete's left side while I positioned myself on his right in order to stabilize his humerus against his thorax as we got him up and walked him off the field.

The athlete only took about 3 steps when, suddenly, his legs began to buckle. He was about to experience syncope, possibly as a result of hypovolemic shock. As we lowered the athlete back to the ground, that same adrenalin rush I had felt when I first confirmed the diagnosis had returned, albeit this time accompanied by equal amounts of terror. What had I done? Why didn't I take the advice of the coach and summon the EMS personnel onto the field?

In an effort to rectify the mistake I had made and redeem myself for the sake of this injured athlete, I focused on assessing his condition and making certain not to exacerbate the injury. Luckily, the athlete did not lose consciousness and he remained alert throughout. Once it was established that the injured athlete was stable enough to triage appropriately, I summoned the EMS personnel who assisted me in applying a splint to the fractured arm. The athlete was placed on a gurney and into the ambulance for transport to the emergency room. The athlete later underwent surgery to stabilize the fracture with a plate and screws and his subsequent recovery was, thankfully, unremarkable.

REFLECTION

As I reflected on this incident, there were several assumptions I had mistakenly made that could have been detrimental to this athlete's well-being. First, the athlete's calm demeanor gave me the false sense that this injury did not pose the sort of threat or could rise to the level of severity that I should have recognized it to be. Perhaps worse though, was the degree of hubris I demonstrated in thinking that I could manage this injury like any typical orthopedic injury I had encountered previously. This was a very humbling realization, but it served as a powerful learning experience for me that positively impacted my decision making as my career progressed. It also serves as a reminder to never take any such similar situation for granted and that an effective clinician is one who puts the safety and care of the patient first, utilizing all the resources available to achieve the desired outcome.

HEY REF!

Marirose Radelet, MS, PT, LAT, ATC

KEY TERMS

Helmet-to-Helmet Hit | Concussion | Referee Calls

Community sponsored midget football leagues operate from July through late October or November with playoffs and championship rounds. The leagues are open to boys and girls ages 5 to 14. Many of the leagues are registered as not-for-profit with the state. Each group raises its own funding for the year through registration fees, concession stand sales, hoagie, popcorn and various other sales. Each group usually operates under the umbrella of one organization whose board of directors consists of one member from each league. The organization sets and enforces the rules for all leagues, schedules the games, and determines the outcomes of disputes between leagues. The organization hires and assigns referees for each game. Each league is responsible for paying the referees and security at each of their home games. There are no emergency medical services personnel at games. Emergencies are handled by calling 911 and waiting for the first available transport. During the first game of the season, a deliberate helmet-to-knee hit fractured a player's kneecap and he was out for the season.

TRUE STORY #7

During a tightly contested Saturday regulation game between 2 13- to 14-year-old league teams, there were 2 helmet-to-helmet hits within 10 minutes, both resulting in offensive players injured on the field. The first athlete was supine and conscious but did not move and was slow to respond to verbal questions. He complained of a headache and dizziness. He was oriented to time and place, but did not know what happened to him. He could actively move all extremities when instructed, although his response to instructions was slow. He showed slight nystagmus following left to right finger movements in his left eye. After a few minutes, his dizziness had decreased. He was assisted to a sitting position where he continued to complain of a headache and dizziness. After a brief time he was assisted off the field by 2 coaches. He showed ataxic gait and poor balance while walking to the sideline. The athletic trainer determined that he should be transported to the nearest emergency department and had security contact his family in the stands to transport him there. There referee did not call a penalty for the hit.

The second helmet-to-helmet hit resulted in another offensive player down on the field. Once again, the referee failed to indicate a penalty. The player was conscious and crying, stating he had been hit in the head by a helmet and had a headache. He was responsive to verbal commands, could move all extremities, and was oriented to time and place. The referee was observing the assessment closely. The athletic trainer looked up at him and said, "Are you going to call any of this? This is the second helmet-to-helmet hit in 10 minutes."

The referee said, "You take care of your kid. I'll take care of the field." The athletic trainer continued assessing the player and then had him assisted off the field.

"You're going to get someone killed."

The referee replied, "You take care of your business. I'll take care of mine."

The following Monday, that group of referees was terminated from organization participation.

REFLECTION

After the injured athletes were taken care of, I calmed down and thought about the situation. I realized that the referees may have had the authority to throw me out of the game. If that had happened, there would not have been any medical personnel on the field for either team for the rest of the day; however, if the referees didn't start calling violations for these blatant helmet-to-helmet hits, someone might be killed. I realized that unintentional helmet-to-helmet hits happen in football. but the referees hired by the specific inner city minority organization we belonged to seemed to have a high tolerance for violence on the field. Coaches throughout the leagues knew what the rules were but seemed to allow their players to engage in dangerous tackling practices so long as a penalty wasn't called. This question remains, do I, as an athletic trainer, have the right or the obligation to speak to referees about situations that endanger the athletes?

It gave me some satisfaction to find out the next week that that group of referees was terminated from organization participation. I also questioned my actions concerning injured athlete number one. Should he have been walked off the field for family transport to the emergency department or should an ambulance have been called to the field to transport him? Given the lengthy response time for city emergency medical services units and his off-field assessment, I believe I would make the same decision in future similar situations. His postinjury ImPACT (ImPact Applications, Inc.) test, given during the next week, showed scores that were not significantly different from his baseline test.

Guns at the Field

Marirose Radelet, MS, PT, LAT, ATC

Key Terms

Football Practice | Shooting | Safety Policies

A majority of community-sponsored urban midget football leagues in Western Pennsylvania practice on public fields. These leagues are open to boys and girls ages 5 to 14. Teams are assembled by age group. In general, every football and cheerleading team practices on the same field at the same time (4 to 5 evenings per week). For the league described in this story, the field space included a public basketball court that was used by older teens during the same early evening hours as practice.

True Story #8

During a regular midget football league evening practice in the middle of July, a fight broke out between 2 16-year-olds on the basketball court adjacent to the field. Two of the football coaches went over to try to calm things down between the teens. The coaches left the basketball court thinking that the dispute had been resolved. Unfortunately, 2 of the teens went to their cars, got their guns, and began firing at each other. The gunshots continued for several minutes leaving one of the teens gravely wounded and one of the league cheerleaders wounded in the knee. There was panic on the football field with parents covering kids with their bodies or grabbing their kids and running away.

Reflection

This did not happen to my league but to a league in the same area of the city; however, I was deeply affected by it. I feel like I am responsible for the safety of the children in my league. We have had a gunshot policy in our emergency action plan and standard operating procedure for the last 10 years. It is based on the recommendations of the police at that time and states that in case of gunshots, every adult present should yell, "GET DOWN, GET DOWN, GET DOWN," and enforce the action without putting themselves at risk. But should these recommendations change from 10 years ago now that guns seem to be the urban way of settling disputes?

In the week following the shootings the community stepped forward to support the league. The parents were determined that the league would continue. The police pledged daily presence at the field for 2 weeks then an increased patrol presence, money was raised for private security, and a discussion with the city concerning shutting down the basketball court during football practice took place.

Concerned about my own league safety, I contacted the local police, first responders, and local emergency medical technicians about the recommended action when gunshots occur during football events. They had no definitive recommendations. The commander of our police zone said we should do whatever we feel would make our participants safe.

At a parent and coaches meeting, our league decided to stay with the same action plan that is outlined in our emergency action plan/standard operating procedure.

HE HAS WHAT?

Robert O. Blanc, MS, LAT, ATC, EMT-P

KEY TERMS

Multiple Sclerosis | Neurologic Findings | Differential Diagnosis

The role of the athletic trainer has changed dramatically over the years. The education that we receive is extensive, and the science and technology that we have access to is amazing; however, just when you think you have a solid grasp on things, something occurs that proves you wrong. The only way to overcome these situations is to build a strong system by which you can offer the best care: physical, mental and emotional. Don't be afraid to build strong relationships in the community and rely on others who may have more expertise in an area. That is what separates the good athletic trainers from the great ones.

TRUE STORY #9

I had been the head athletic trainer at a Division I school for 6 years, had worked with a National Football League (NFL) team for 5 years and been through well-known undergraduate and graduate athletic training programs. I had a strong background in emergency medical services and therefore felt very confident that I was ready for anything that athletic training could hand me. I had dealt with shoulder dislocations, a tibia/fibula fracture, anterior cruciate ligament tears and just about any other "sports injury" you could imagine. As a paramedic, I had seen just about everything else, motor vehicle accidents, falls from heights, sick children, suicides, and much more. My confidence in my ability to handle any situation was very high. I had been trained by some of the best people in their fields.

The game was in Florida in early October and was unusually hot for us northerners. We had some issues with the heat but other than that we had a pretty clean game injury-wise. In the middle of the third quarter, our quarterback threw an interception. On the return, one of our offensive linemen was pursuing to make the tackle and got "clothes lined" on the far sideline. We made our way over to him, stabilized his head and our team physician proceeded with his evaluation. He described a "stinger" with an electric feeling going down his left arm immediately but it dissipated shortly after we had begun evaluating him. The only other finding was anterior neck pain where he had been hit. There weren't any significant neurologic findings other than some slight weakness in his left bicep, and there wasn't any cervical pain. He said he was ok so he sat up, stood, and made his way to our sideline.

Upon further evaluation, there were no other findings. He regained full strength, had full range of motion, no signs of traumatic brain injury and stated that he felt fine. After a long discussion on the sideline, the athlete admitted to having "many" stingers which were unreported. Our team physician felt that we should get X-rays as a precaution which were available at the stadium. The X-rays were normal and he was cleared to return to the game. He finished the game without incident, but after the game he complained of having some stiffness in his neck and his throat was sore from the collision. He did not report any trouble breathing, swallowing, or speaking.

Sunday treatments are always a mystery. You never know what might show up, injuries that occurred on Saturday that you didn't know about. This was a fairly typical Sunday from that sense. We saw an ankle sprain, rib contusion, nothing we couldn't handle. Our lineman came in feeling pretty good, still stiff with slightly less range of motion than Saturday, but nothing alarming. His strength was equal bilaterally and there weren't any other neurologic findings. Upon further questioning regarding his recurrent stingers, he had had them since high school. They were transient in nature, usually occurring on his left side and never evaluated. He didn't think it was anything to be concerned about.

We decided that magnetic resonance imaging (MRI) was needed to truly determine what was going on, and so we scheduled him for that Monday. The athlete wasn't happy about the idea, mostly because he had to get up early on his off day to get the scan; however, he begrudgingly agreed to get the MRI even though he didn't think it was necessary.

Monday evening our team physician called with the results. The diagnosis was multiple sclerosis (MS). I asked the doctor to repeat the results about 3 times before it sunk in. This was one of the biggest, strongest, healthiest young men on our team. He was projected to be a high NFL draft pick and now was facing a dreadful diagnosis. I didn't sleep that night, or many subsequent nights. I wondered how we were going to break this news to him. This was not in any book I had read or any conference I had attended.

The following morning, I met with the team physician and we talked about how to proceed. We were part of a large hospital system and had amazing resources. We contacted the neurology department and were able to reach the head of the department who specialized in treating MS. He agreed to take this case on himself.

The athlete showed up for treatment that morning and the team physician and I met with him and went over the findings. As you would expect he was sure that the results were wrong, after all he had never had any symptoms and was perfectly healthy. We assured him that it had been caught early in its development and that there were new treatments that he would have access to. We contacted his mother and explained things to her as well. The neurologist had agreed to see him the following day; I accompanied him to that appointment. The doctor explained in great detail what was going on and talked about the options and prognosis which were promising at the time. He was to begin a regimen of interferon treatments immediately. The goal was to limit the disease's progression and symptoms and allow him to live a "normal" life for as long as possible. Of course, the question of football came up quickly. The doctor said that there wasn't any literature on people playing football with documented cases of MS, but he didn't see why he couldn't if he wasn't having symptoms. This came as a huge relief to the athlete.

He began the treatments and had no side effects from them. He continued to train and perform as he had always done without difficulties. We monitored him very closely. As time went on we noticed that he would fatigue more quickly than previously, but he would alert us to that and we adjusted his activities accordingly.

He appeared to handle the situation very well. He seemed to go about his life as he had before the diagnosis. Teammates hadn't noticed any changes in him nor had the coaching staff. Things were going well, or so I thought. Over the next few months the athlete failed 3 university drug tests and was disqualified from the team and lost his scholarship. He was placed in a rehab program immediately after the first positive test and remained there until his dismissal. He transferred to another university where he played for one year. He was given a tryout by one NFL team but was cut shortly after.

I have not seen or heard from this athlete since shortly after he left us. I often wonder how he is doing and what his life has offered him.

REFLECTION

There isn't a textbook with advice on having to tell a young, healthy individual that they have a disease that could change their life. We learn to identify injuries and immediately work to return athletes to their sport. I never imagined that this would be something that I would have to deal with. Since then, I have had to deal with many health issues that had nothing to do with athletics. Discussing lymphoma, diabetes, enlarged hearts and aortic aneurysm are not easy conversations to have with young, healthy individuals. As an athletic trainer, these individuals trust you and rely on you to protect them. It is a feeling that you will experience unlike anything you have experienced before, absolute helplessness.

Unfortunately, a similar situation is probably going to happen to you at some point in your professional career. Your instincts will be to find a way to heal them as you have so many anterior cruciate ligaments, ankle sprains, and broken bones. I think it is important to attack any diagnosis with this attitude but know that you can't always fix everything.

I often wonder if I did enough to help this young man deal with his diagnosis, especially in terms of mental health. What could I have done to encourage a more positive outlook on things and prevent him from losing his scholarship and continue to work toward his dreams? I now think about these things whenever any athlete gets injured or sick. It is the whole athlete that we must rehabilitate.

Domain II

Clinical Evaluation
and Diagnosis

THIS WASN'T IN THE TEXTBOOK

James Cerullo, PhD, ATC, CSCS

KEY TERMS

Entrance Wound | Femur | Fracture

I came upon the profession of athletic training indirectly. Despite having played high school sports, I had never even entered an athletic training room. All I knew about our trainer, Al, was that he smoked a cigar and walked with a limp. I believe he had a prosthetic leg.

After graduating high school, I studied business administration for 2 years at Massachusetts Bay Community College. I was certain of 2 things: I did not want to sit behind a desk 8 hours a day, and I wanted to play college football. After the dean of students called me into her office to explain it would take me 3 years to get a two-year degree, I transferred to Westfield State College. By doing so, I transitioned from club football to National Collegiate Athletic Association Division III. Unfortunately, when I received my academic schedule: anatomy and physiology, kinesiology and introduction to athletic training, I knew my dream of football was over.

I wanted to stay involved in sports; I felt this strongly. Following the suggestion of my academic advisor, I talked to Westfield's head trainer. After I introduced myself, he handed me a telephone and a Cramer black metal first aid kit. He told me where the phone jack was and asked me to cover field hockey practice, and I should call him if something were to happen.

He had more confidence in me than I had in myself. I thought he was crazy, but I ended up covering my first practice as an athletic training student and over the next 3 years covered a variety of practices, preseason camps, and games. At that time, in order to sit for the national certification exam, I had to log 1800 hours. Eventually, I achieved this. By any standard, my career has been a full one and includes 11 years of college, 3 degrees, and 2 national certifications. It started with a little more than a handshake, a rotary telephone, a field hockey practice, and a first aid kit. It started with an impulse and instinctual desire.

Gorse KM, Feld F, Blanc RO, eds.
True Stories From the Athletic Training Room (pp 33-57).
© 2018 SLACK Incorporated.

TRUE STORY #10

I remember my interview into the doctoral program at the University of Pittsburgh (Pitt). The director of the graduate athletic training curriculum was blunt in his feelings towards classes. As a doctoral student, you were there to do research. This man would serve as my dissertation advisor. His guidance and patience would be instrumental in helping me complete my degree.

My assistantship would be with the football team. This was a Division I football program with a rich history of sending players into the National Football League (NFL). Some of these players, such as Mike Ditka and Tony Dorsett, would go on to storied professional careers and be inducted into both the College Football and Professional Football Hall of Fame. I remember watching this particular team on television in 1976 and reading about Tony Dorsett winning the Heisman Trophy in *Sports Illustrated*. It was hard to believe 11 years removed from my undergraduate degree, I was a graduate assistant athletic trainer for the same college football program I had read about when I was in junior high school. Immediately I started to question my abilities. What was I doing here? Did I deserve to be here? The rigor of a doctoral program in sports medicine would be enough of a challenge. The addition of being a graduate assistant staff athletic trainer with the added responsibilities of being at every preseason camp, practice, and game was overwhelming. I was older than every other graduate student in the program. Most had gone straight through from an undergraduate into a graduate program. There was maybe one or 2 who had worked a year or 2 in the profession and then decided to pursue a graduate degree. By comparison, I was an old man. One of the younger graduate students had even nicknamed me Uncle Jimmy."

The first practice I covered in Pitt Football Stadium upon our return from preseason camp found me in a pair of Nike (Nike Inc.) sneakers despite our Adidas (Adidas AG) sponsorship. Our head athletic director came by to watch practice, saw my footwear and had a few choice words for the equipment manager, after which the equipment manager and I sprinted off the field so he could fit me with a pair of Adidas turf shoes.

The first year was a challenge physically, emotionally, and intellectually. It was vital to gain the trust not only of the full-time staff athletic trainers and team physicians, but also, and more importantly, the players. Being a graduate assistant meant that everything I did had to be communicated back to Rob, the head trainer and Kevin, his assistant. They, in turn, had to deal with the coaching staff which could be stressful at times.

I remember my first opportunity to perform an ankle evaluation. It wasn't a serious injury and the evaluation took place after practice in the training room. Over the course of 10 years, I had done these countless times and felt confident in my skills; however, my confidence was shattered within seconds of placing Vernon's ankle in what I thought was the proper limb positioning as it had been taught to me by Doc, one of our team physicians. He proceeded to correct me immediately. A knowing smirk came across Vernon's face as Doc started to quote several journal articles citing specific titles and dates and why the textbooks were wrong and why I was wrong too.

I was deflated. It took me weeks until I mustered enough courage to attempt another evaluation. Despite this, at the end of my first year, I asked Doc if he would be willing to serve on my dissertation committee. After all, he was a living, breathing, encyclopedic, walking Medline. He saved me many trips to the medical school library and had read from the mountains of journal articles stacked in his office.

It took me this whole first year to get settled into a routine and adapt to living on a graduate assistant stipend. There were countless times when I would question my abilities as an athletic trainer. Fortunately, Rob the head athletic trainer, along with orthopedic fellows, provided some needed comic relief from the grind of my academic studies. Collectively, they assumed the role of matchmaker and felt responsible for finding a love connection for me. Unfortunately, this backfired and I found myself unwillingly playing the role of matchmaker for a vivacious cheerleader. Rob and the rest of the sports medicine staff took great joy in watching this unfold.

There were others who helped me out too, such as Buddy Morris, our head strength coach. Buddy had a colorful vocabulary and my first interaction with him was unplanned. The collegiate football season was over and the NFL was beginning their postseason playoffs. During this time, players who had been drafted from the University of Pittsburgh football program would come back to campus specifically to train with Buddy as they prepared for the next season. On this particular day, there were half a dozen of them standing in the lounge adjacent to the weight room discussing their workouts with Buddy. The combined weight of the men in that room was well over 1800 pounds with an average height of 6 feet, 4 inches. At the time, I weighed about 165 pounds. I was half the size of the next smallest guy in the room.

I had to enter the room to get a textbook I had left on the table. As I walked in, Buddy turned to me and in front of these NFL players who were built like steel girders with heads. Cursing, he said, "I hate doctoral students." The players glared at me. The room went silent. Buddy spoke again referring to me, "But he's okay." To this day I'm not sure what I did, but I'm glad Buddy had such kind words for me.

In the 3 years' time, I had exciting experiences, was immersed in cutting edge sports medicine, and had the pleasure of working with highly respected professors, doctors, and athletic trainers. I remember the day I defended my dissertation. Doc and Rob were there sitting in the back of the room, the former because he had to and the latter for moral support. My defense went well. A handful of questions were asked, which I answered adequately. When it was over, I walked out into an empty hallway. I looked right. No one. I looked left. Still no one. I remember thinking—is this it? Prior to the start of my defense, I had noticed Rob lean over and whisper something to Doc. I found out later that Rob had told Doc to go easy on me. I remain forever grateful to Rob for this.

Several weeks later I moved to New York to begin a position as director for the athletic training education program at Alfred University. After 4 years as a program director dealing with the bureaucracy of accreditation, I left Alfred. I accepted a position as assistant professor of athletic training at Grand Valley State University in Western Michigan. After 5 years, I began to realize that perhaps teaching and academia were not a good fit. I missed the clinical aspect of being on the playing field. I missed the camaraderie, emotion, and intensity. This was a difficult time for me. Then something happened.

Rob called me and asked how I was doing. I told him the truth that I was ready for a change. Rob then told me that his assistant was leaving and asked if I was interested in coming back to the University of Pittsburgh to work with him. My first response was, "You're joking?" I had a tremendous amount of respect for Rob and told him I'd drop everything for an opportunity to work with him again. When he realized I was serious, we discussed my salary. Several days later I was on campus for a formal interview. I met with the head football coach. When he saw all the certifications after my name, he had only one question, "Do you know how to tape an ankle?" Thus began my second stint with the Pitt football program, but this time as a full-time assistant.

It was late June and summer conditioning had started. Most of the Pitt players were already on campus and Rob needed me there in 2 weeks. I gave my notice at Grand Valley State, packed a suitcase and spent the next 2 days driving to the football complex. Packing and moving the rest of my belongings would have to wait. Most of the coaches who were on staff during my graduate assistant days had been fired or moved on to new positions, but some had survived the head coaching changes over the years and were still on staff. This included our director of football operations and defensive backs' coach. Doc was still there and so was Ox, the equipment manager. Pitt's new head football coach, the man who had interviewed me, had just completed his first year. He was talking about bringing back Buddy who had left to work for the Cleveland Browns. My first week back I remember sitting down with Doc to review magnetic resonance imaging images of injured players who had needed surgery. I learned more from Doc in 20 minutes than I had during the past 5 years.

Back at Pitt, I had no delusions about what my primary role would be. I was there to make Rob's job easier. My responsibilities would be to oversee the rehabilitation protocols so Rob could manage the daily operational procedures and administrative duties. I minimized my doctorate degree and never brought it up in conversation. This changed when the football media guide was published. What was a PhD in sports medicine doing on the sidelines covering football practice? Most athletic trainers I knew who went back for a PhD did so to get off the field and not have to work 15 hour days, 7 days a week. It took me about a month to settle in. My taping skills were a bit rusty, but after taping 12 ankles a day, twice a day for 3 months they quickly returned.

August arrived and preseason camp began. The coaches began to say, "We're doing it for real." As a trainer, I had to be "on" all the time. Once camp ended, I'd get into a weekly routine.

Pitt won 5 out of 11 games, a losing season. There was talk of coaching changes. The day after the season ended, *The Pittsburgh Tribune Review* jumped all over the story: "Coaching Changes to Be Made." I read the article. Our head coach was quoted saying, "We are going to evaluate our entire staff including the athletic trainers." I asked Rob, "Do we still have jobs?" He didn't know. Anything could happen. In the end, some coaches were fired and some resigned before they could be. Rob and I learned through the team's sports psychologist, who had consulted with the head coach, that we still had jobs.

The fall semester ended. Our jobs were secure for another season. The players went home for their winter break. Approximately 2 weeks before the team was scheduled to return from break and begin winter conditioning workouts, Chris, the director of Pitt football operations, came to see Rob and I. He had serious news. Nick, a defensive tackle, had been shot at home visiting his family in Miami, Florida. While in Miami X-rays had been taken. It was determined that no fractures were present. Nick had been prescribed some antibiotics and pain medication, placed on crutches, and sent home. I was a bit shocked by this. I'd never known anyone who'd been shot, but I'd assumed such a victim would be kept overnight in the hospital as a precaution. Rob and I were now responsible for Nick's rehabilitation and treatment. I would be overseeing his rehab and I was nervous about this. "This wasn't in the textbook. I don't remember learning about this in my care and prevention class," I said to Rob. Rob just shook his head in disbelief.

On his first day of treatment, Nick hobbled on crutches into the training room. He was clutching a folder that contained a copy of his X-rays and home care instructions. These had been given to him by the attending emergency room physician in Miami. Nick, nonplussed, hopped onto one of the treatment tables and rolled-up the pant leg of his sweats. The entrance wound had already started to heal and there appeared to be no obvious signs of infection. The bullet had entered the lateral side of his thigh above the knee and stopped midway through the distal femur. He told Rob and me that because the bullet was from a small caliber hand gun the Miami doctors had decided to leave it in place.

We took his X-rays into the exam room and placed them on the light box. There it was, a small fragment about the size of a pencil eraser lodged in the distal femur several inches above the lateral epicondyle.

I turned to Rob, "I don't know the first thing about treating a gunshot wound." He replied, "Just follow the instructions given by the emergency room physician. There's no fracture. Treat it like a thigh contusion." We then discussed a treatment plan. Although Nick wasn't listed as a first team defensive tackle, he had started more than several games the previous season and was used often as a situational substitute. One of the first questions he asked was if he would be ready for spring ball. At this point, I deferred to Rob who told Nick it would be a day-to-day process.

The next morning, which would mark the first official day of Nick's rehabilitation, he came into the training room still on crutches but able to partially bear weight on his injured leg. He was highly motivated, as most Division I football players are, and immediately wanted to get started. I pulled his file and started a rehab log sheet. The initial prescription called for range of motion exercises and standard wound care. We began with basic heel slides followed by ankle pumps. I cleaned and dressed his wound and ended the session with 20 minutes on the Game Ready (CoolSystems). The next day, Doc evaluated his injured leg to make sure the entrance wound was healing. We progressed accordingly adding standard exercises for a combination knee-thigh injury. I continued to follow the original treatment instructions and by the end of the first week Nick was able to pedal on the stationary bike to approximately 90 degrees at the knee of his injured leg. He attempted to complete a full revolution, but couldn't control his quadriceps. Still, I thought he was making remarkable progress.

After 2 weeks of daily rehab sessions, with the help of some slight lateral trunk flexion, Nick was able to complete a full revolution on the bike using his injured leg. During this time, Rob and I consulted with Doc about Nick's progress. We agreed a new set of X-rays was warranted.

Doc called in the order. The morning following the X-rays, Rob told me, "You're not going to believe this. Doc is on his way over." As Rob completed this sentence Doc burst into the room. We followed him into the exam room and watched as he logged into his hospital account and pulled up the most recent X-rays. There on the computer screen was a fractured femur. Nick's leg was broken and several inches above the bullet his femur was shattered and displaced. A callus was visible where some healing had already begun. Doc explained that the radiologist he'd consulted with had called in all his residents and interns to lecture them on the importance of taking images of the entire limb, not just the entrance wound. No one had told Nick about these latest X-rays or the open reduction procedure that would come next. His football career was over.

REFLECTION

I spent the remainder of the semester ruminating over Nick's career-ending injury. How had I not seen this? As an undergraduate, I had learned in a first aid course about the signs and symptoms of a femur fracture. I felt awful. Rob and Doc had assured me that I'd done nothing wrong. Collectively, we had followed care instructions based on how the initial X-ray had been read and there wasn't a fracture. In addition, after 2 weeks of treatment and over 6 weeks since the incident, Nick hadn't progressed as expected. Our medical team had made the correct diagnosis. Countless conversations ensued between us, but I couldn't let it go. I felt like I acted unprofessionally and lost more than one night's sleep over it.

About this time, a colleague recommended Malcolm Gladwell's book, *Blink*. Although Mr. Gladwell doesn't like the term, "blink" refers to listening to one's gut instinct. As I read, I thought back to the day when I'd witnessed Nick's leg flopping on the treatment table. At that time, I'd dismissed this, intent on following instructions from the original emergency room physician in Miami. After finishing Gladwell's book, I began to recall episodes in my life as an athletic trainer when a thought had entered my mind and I had pushed it aside labeling it as unreasonable. These days, I tell my students that 90 percent of their diagnostic skills will come from their ability to take a thorough medical history, while at the same time listening intently to a patient's responses. The remaining 10 percent comes from listening to one's instincts. In addition to the classic, *Principles of Athletic Training,* I believe Gladwell's *Blink* should be required reading for all athletic training students. Why? Because sometimes the best answers aren't found in the textbook.

A COMPLETE KNEE DISLOCATION

Peggy A. Houglum, PhD

In an emergency, having a plan in place ahead of time is vital to providing an optimal outcome. People involved in emergency care must be calm, level-headed, and prepared for any injury, working as a team for the injured individual. Luck can be an additional blessing that provides the individual with a happy ending of a near-disastrous event.

TRUE STORY #11

While working at the Olympic Training Center in Colorado Springs, Colorado, I was assigned to a wrestling competition. On a day of competition, I was sitting on the sidelines with an orthopedist when a participant was lifted and flipped into the air by his opponent. As he landed, his foot stuck into the mat. The impact force of the drop caused his tibia to dislocate posteriorly on his femur. The physician and I quickly went to his side. As I tried to calm and reassure the athlete, the physician performed the emergency examination. It was obvious that the knee was fully dislocated; the tibia was positioned far ahead of the femur and the patient was in severe pain and unable to move his foot. The physician palpated for a popliteal pulse and reported that it was present. He also examined for possible fracture. While other medical support personnel called for an ambulance, we splinted the knee and continued to monitor for a pulse and watch for signs of shock.

Emergency medical technicians quickly arrived, and the athlete was transported to the emergency department of the local hospital. Once in the hospital, it was discovered that there was no popliteal pulse, and he was rushed into the operating room.

The athlete was fortunate on 2 counts: 1) a microvascular surgeon happened to be present in the hospital at the time and was able to save the limb by restoring the damaged blood vessels; and 2) a world-renowned orthopedic surgeon was visiting the

Olympic Training Center during this time. He was contacted and performed surgery on the ruptured knee ligaments to restore stability to the knee.

Although the athlete was informed that he would never participate in athletics again, after extensive rehabilitation, he returned to running. He was thankful that his leg was not amputated and was able to resume some sport activities.

REFLECTION

Rapid response to an emergency situation with the luck of the presence of a microvascular surgeon and expert orthopedist saved the leg of this athlete. Had any of these elements of care not been present, the positive outcome he experienced would not have occurred.

ALWAYS FIND OUT WHAT THEY ARE DOING IN THEIR OFF TIME

Mary Mundrane-Zweiacher, PT, ATC, CHT

KEY TERMS

Overuse | Flexor Carpi Ulnaris | Detailed History

When evaluating patients and athletes, they often tell you what they feel is significant and subconsciously rule out that there could be other factors causing their condition. Athletic trainers sometimes need to be more persistent in their questioning to ensure that they have the most accurate history and causative factors.

TRUE STORY #12

A college lacrosse athlete came into the athletic training room complaining of right ulnar wrist pain. It was March and basically the middle of lacrosse season. He had no mechanism of injury that he could think of and did not have problems with his right wrist or upper extremity before. During questioning, he said he had not sustained a fall or played longer than usual and was not doing anything different. The pain progressively increased during a 2 week period and it was becoming difficult for him to take a shot on goal. He experienced pain while attempting to ulnarly deviate and flex the right wrist but range of motion was generally equal bilaterally. He was also found to have muscle weakness, especially with manual muscle testing to the flexor carpi ulnaris (FCU). Upon palpation, he had tenderness with thickening over the right FCU, pisiform, hook of the hamate and base of the fifth metacarpal (volar aspect).

The assessment was that he had FCU tendinitis and treatment was initiated. In conjunction with the team physician, this player was put on anti-inflammatories and given treatment in the athletic training room. Treatment in the athletic training room consisted of ultrasound, soft tissue massage to the distal FCU, range of motion stretching within pain-free limits, pain-free strengthening, and Bodyblade exercise. High-voltage electrical stimulation was also performed with cold pack after treatment for pain and swelling relief. The athlete was also put in a wrist cock-up splint to rest the right wrist musculature and practice was modified. His pain complaints were only intermittently relieved and his pain scale would sometimes go back to his evaluation level. It was 2 weeks into his rehabilitation without significant improvement when I heard him talking about his part-time job. I asked him what his job was and he told me he was a scooper and mixer at an ice cream shop. This a shop where customers pick things like gummy bears, M&Ms (Mars, Incorporated), and other candy that they would like in their ice cream. The employee uses a scraper on cold marble, pulling the ice cream and "add-ins" to mix it all together. Kinesthetically, this action is primarily done by the FCU, with contributions from the flexor digitorum superficialis, flexor digitorum profundus, triceps, posterior deltoid, and some latissimus dorsi. With further questioning, he shared that he worked as many hours as he could around his lacrosse schedule so he worked often during the week but primarily on the weekend. He had just started this part-time job this spring semester but did not think it was significant. I had a discussion with the athlete about overuse conditions and the need for muscles to rest from excessive activity. It was mutually concluded that he would stop working at this part-time job until the end of the lacrosse season. Therapy continued in the athletic training room and this athlete was able to resume play without limitation after approximately one week.

REFLECTION

When patients or athletes come to a medical professional to treat a problem, they have often done some internal analysis and may have a bias as to what they think are the causative or precipitating factors. No athletic trainer or therapist has an infinite amount of time and while there may be some comprehensive questioning during a physical exam, it is equally important to continue asking questions regarding a patient's medical history during the treatment process if the athlete or patient is not making sufficient progress. This athlete did not consider a part-time job in an ice cream shop as a potentially limiting factor, but when he wasn't progressing, the athletic trainer continued to assess the problem to find the solution. When the physical demands of this job were uncovered, it was understandable why flexor carpi ulnaris tendinitis developed.

WHEN TAKING A MEDICAL HISTORY, DON'T ASSUME

Michael Hanley, ATC, LAT

KEY TERMS

Medical History | Clinical Evaluation | Clinical Experience

I was taught during my athletic training education that obtaining a thorough medical history was the most important aspects of the clinical examination. This was stressed over many years of athletic training practice to the point where accurate clinical impressions could be formed simply from the history. Having an idea of what an injury might be helped guide the hands-on examination process, which might be important in helping reduce the length of time it took to complete the evaluation. When an athlete complained of only medial knee pain and related a valgus force as a mechanism, the clinician could, with a good degree of confidence, deduce that the medial collateral ligament was involved. With an absence of lateral pain and a defined mechanism, one could save time focusing on things other than varus stress testing, lateral joint line exam, muscle testing, and similar tests. With time being of the essence in a hectic postpractice athletic training room, saving precious minutes by eliminating needless tests make for a more efficient evaluation process. Twenty years of athletic training experience reinforced my belief. One day changed it.

TRUE STORY #13

Our athletic training department utilizes the services of a sports medicine fellow provided by our university medical school. The upside of this is obvious as we have the ability to profit from another licensed physician in the health care of our student athletes. The downside is that these fellows are usually quite inexperienced in athletically related problems, and the college-aged population in general, and the learning curve in developing proper evaluation skills can be quite steep.

The first fellow we ever had was a family practice physician who wanted to develop the skills and experience necessary to become a team physician at the college or professional level. The majority of his day was spent at his general medicine practice, evaluating patients ranging from the very young to the very old, with occasional opportunities to deal with athletic injuries, particularly those of an orthopedic nature. He would then come over to the athletic training room in the afternoons and see the 18- to 22-year-old population exclusively with injuries and conditions almost universally related to participation in sports.

At the beginning of his fellowship, watching him perform an evaluation was almost painful. He would ask medical history questions that appeared more relevant to the elderly patients at his clinic than to the college-aged patients in our athletic training room. There were many times when I wanted to step in and try to steer him back on track as he veered into questions that seemed unrelated to the problem of the student athlete sitting in front of him. I was pretty sure that the football player being evaluated after having been struck in the ribs by a helmet wasn't currently under care for tuberculosis, but the fellow was so used to asking those types of questions that it was second nature to him. Meanwhile, his patient schedule would run behind as he took extra time to make the same diagnosis that the athletic trainer had made almost immediately upon exam on the field. Every student athlete brought in with dizziness and lightheadedness has almost always experienced some sort of cardiac event, at least until it was determined that they hadn't eaten all day and hadn't hydrated at practice. Because of our experiences, the athletic trainers knew right away what the problem was. I can clearly recall the fellow asking whether or not the student athlete had chest pain, back pain, pain radiating into the neck left arm, tightness in the chest, trouble breathing, and the like. Which, if you've ever examined a player right after practice, the answer to most of those is yes. It took a while, but the fellow eventually got the hang of it. He became very skilled at exams and history-taking. While he never stopped asking cardiac-based questions when examining student athletes with chest discomfort (and I gave up trying to convince him he was wasting his time asking), he eventually discovered that in the population of young, healthy, college student athletes, the simplest answer to a problem is usually the correct one.

With that as a preface, my true story involves an athlete (I will refer to him as TC) who came in for evaluation of fatigue and mild chest discomfort after running during an offseason workout in February. He was a 21-year-old African American with a recent past medical history significant for gastroenteritis followed by a upper respiratory infection (URI) and allergy symptoms within the 3 to 4 weeks prior to the onset of his current complaints. The symptoms of his URI included productive cough and tightness in his chest. He had been withheld from activity during his illnesses. He was known to be hypertensive and denied taking any medications or supplements.

During the exam in the athletic training room, TC related mild retrosternal pain. He described this pain as similar to the discomfort he experienced during with his previous cough. He denied shortness of breath. His blood pressure was 160/94 and was pulse was 84. His breath sounded normal. After cooling off, his symptoms began to subside. I called the team physician, who felt this was related to the previous URI. He agreed to see him the next morning if symptoms persisted. For some reason, before discharging TC, I recalled the advice our fellow always gave to our student athletes with similar symptoms—the advice I always thought was a waste of time. I told TC that if he should develop any increased chest pain, back pain, or radiating pain into his neck or left arm that he should call me.

Two hours later, my phone rang. It was TC. He had begun developing some pain in the upper left side of his back. He denied worsening of any of the symptoms he had exhibited after the workout. I picked him up at his apartment and drove him to the hospital still convinced that this was URI related. Upon arrival at the emergency room, an electrocardiogram was performed and read as normal. Lab work revealed some slightly elevated cardiac enzymes. The working diagnosis became likely pericarditis, with the thought that this was triggered by his previous illnesses. After some discussion, the treating physician elected to perform a cardiac catheterization to rule out more significant causes of TC's discomfort. After the physician walked out of the exam room, the catheterization (cath) technician came in and indicated to me privately that, in her opinion, with her experience of seeing cardiac patients and with her knowledge of TC's case, the procedure was unnecessary. There was no way an otherwise healthy 21-year-old with a normal electrocardiogram and only slightly elevated enzymes had any significant cardiac event. As TC was wheeled into the cath lab, I just hoped that they would be finished fairly quickly.

Shortly into the procedure, the same cath. tech came to find me in the waiting room. They had discovered a large clot at the descending branch of the left anterior coronary artery, otherwise known as a widowmaker block. They were attempting to dissolve it, but she suggested I reach TC's mother because they weren't sure he was going to survive the procedure. I had gone from thinking I was wasting a night in the hospital to making a phone call at 3 o'clock AM informing a mother who lived 3 hours away that she needed to get to the hospital as soon as she could because her son might not live through the night.

Luckily, after 2 separate procedures, they were able to get the clot dissolved. Further testing revealed no structural damage to the heart. It was later determined that TC had multiple heredity factors which predisposed him to clotting. The story eventually had a happy ending. After sitting out for a year, TC was actually able to return to his sport and competed for 2 more years without any issues.

REFLECTION

There are many times when athletic trainers are in a hurry, or tired at the end of a long day. When an athlete comes in with what appears to be a benign condition or problem, it's easy to jump to a conclusion as to what the condition appears to be without taking a complete history or performing a full evaluation. We use our years of experience and skip a question or 2. In most cases, our initial impression is correct and our evaluation method is reinforced.

My experience with TC changed the way I approached clinical exams. Although I could be correct 99 out of 100 times when I use an abbreviated evaluation, the one time I'm wrong might truly be the difference between life and death. TC was in no obvious distress when I evaluated him after his workout. For some reason, and I'll never know why, I remembered the advice our fellow gave to all those patients about signs and symptoms of a cardiac event. I repeated those to TC although I was sure I was wasting time. In one of the many conversations I had with TC's cardiologist, I told him the story about giving TC the signs and symptoms and how I never really included that in my exams before. He told me that by speaking up I most likely saved TC's life as he probably would have died in his sleep that night instead of calling me. I never cut corners on an evaluation after that experience. I never leave a question behind and I certainly have developed a whole new level of respect and patience for our sports medicine fellows.

BEING AN ATHLETIC TRAINER AND FATHER OF A STUDENT ATHLETE

Jeff Shields, MEd, LAT, ATC, CEAS

KEY TERMS

Concussion | ImPACT Test | Concussion Protocol

As a father of 3 multisport high school athletes and a certified athletic trainer for over 30 years, I challenge you to leave your certification at the front door when arriving home from work. There is a reason why physicians do not perform surgery on their family members.

TRUE STORY #14

Kyle, our youngest son made the varsity soccer team as a 5 foot, 7 inch, 125 pound sophomore in high school. He played center midfield and had a very aggressive style of play. He was confident he could win any ball on the ground or in the air. In October 2010, South Central Pennsylvania experienced a week where temperatures were in the high 80s to low 90s with dew points in the 70s. His high school team played 5 games in 8 days in these "summer like" conditions. He started and played significant minutes during games, rarely coming out for a break. After arriving home one evening following this stretch of games, many of which were played on turf fields, Kyle described increased fatigue, general muscle soreness, and a minor headache. He did not report any trauma and said he did not remember any contact or collision to his head or neck region. He also reported that he felt like he was dehydrated during the bus ride home. When Kyle got home he took a quick shower, ate a small meal, drank a few glasses of water and went to bed with a minor headache. He went to school the next day. By when mid-morning he started to feel increased fatigue. The headache became more intense and he started to become sensitive to the bell at the end of classes. Kyle was sent home from school, but performed an ImPACT Test (ImPACT Applications, Inc.) before he came home. All the results were normal when comparing base line numbers. Two days following the onset of symptoms, we took Kyle to a sports medicine physician who helped write the Pennsylvania Interscolastic

Authentic Association concussion protocol and he was diagnosed with a concussion. The first few days following the reported symptoms Kyle experienced difficulty sleeping, loss of appetite, and sensitivity to light and noise. Following the physician visit, was instructed to begin a cocoon period where all stimuli were removed such as phone, computer and listening to music. Following 2 days of the cocoon period, he started to feel much better and many of the symptoms started to disappear. Kyle was placed in the concussion protocol and returned to play without restrictions 16 days postinjury. Kyle wore head gear for the remainder of the high school and travel soccer season. He will be starting his senior season in the fall playing soccer at the college level.

REFLECTION

I was embarrassed and frustrated as a certified athletic trainer that I missed my own son's concussion and relied on my son's reports of dehydration. Health care professionals must remember to be engaged and thorough when evaluating and treating family members.

THINK HORSES, NOT ZEBRAS

Sarah Manspeaker, PhD, LAT, ATC

Conduction of a thorough history, knowledge of pain referral patterns, and awareness of the signs and symptoms of nonorthopedic conditions are vital components of my athletic training evaluation. When patients present with signs and symptoms, it is important to keep the saying, "think horses, not zebras" in mind. This phrase indicates that presenting signs and symptoms will most often lead to a typical diagnosis, a horse, but occasionally an atypical condition may be present, hence the zebra.

TRUE STORY #15

It is late November and basketball season has just commenced with introductory weekend tournaments. The following Monday, a 20-year-old female athlete who completed in the tournament for a competitive Division III program reports to the athletic training clinic following a heavy practice and she is complaining of pain in her right medial thigh, specifically in the proximal third near the adductor group. Given the nature of increased activity during the weekend tournament, the heavy three-point stance focus during practice today, and her 3/5 adductor group manual muscle test on the affected side, the patient is diagnosed with a strain of her adductor group. She is treated with ice for pain and over the next few days begins a gentle stretching and strengthening based rehabilitation program. Within 3 days, all symptoms have resolved, and she has continued to practice and play as normal.

Approximately one month later, the athlete returns from the winter holiday break and begins two-a-day sessions with the team. On the first day back, the team practices for a total of 4 and a half hours. On the second day, the athlete reports that the pain had returned in her right adductor the previous evening, and she took 800 mg of ibuprofen which resolved the pain. When she reports this pain before practice, there is no difference in manual muscle testing score as compared bilaterally, no point tenderness over the adductor group, and no sign of muscle injury. As she is still in pain and wants to practice, the patient takes 600 mg of ibuprofen, goes through gentle stretching and completes practice without incident. Following practice, at which time the athletic trainer has reviewed all prior documentation of this injury, the patient was asked about the timing of her menstrual cycle. The patient indicates that she is due to get her period in approximately 12 days. When shown a calendar dating back to the previous complaint of pain, the athlete indicated that the pain experienced the previous month was also about 13 prior to commencement of her menstrual cycle.

At this time, the athletic trainer discusses the possibility of an ovarian cyst with the athlete and suggests that the patient visit a physician for further evaluation. The patient said that she would contact her parents and discuss this possibility. The patient contacts her parents and her home physician, to whom she states that the symptoms do not hinder her performance or impact her nonathletic aspects of life in a negative way. The physician agrees that an ovarian cyst is a likely cause of her issues and he would like to see her the next time she is home (3 hours away from campus). The next morning, the student, her parents, and the athletic trainer conclude via phone conference that as the athlete is no longer symptomatic, they are willing to wait another month to see if the symptoms occur again prior to scheduling a visit with the physician.

Approximately one month later, the adductor region pain occurs without a direct mechanism or increase in activity level once again. The patient is referred to her physician for evaluation and it is determined through ultrasound that she has a large cyst engulfing her right ovary that is theorized to be referring pain to her medial thigh. The patient elects to complete the remainder of the basketball season (approximately 3 weeks) prior to having the cyst removed. She completes the season without incident.

Upon conclusion of the basketball season, over spring break, the patient undergoes surgical removal of the cyst. The cyst is measured to 8 pounds and equates to the size of a football. The patient returns to basketball conditioning activity 8 weeks following the surgery.

REFLECTION

This case illustrates the important role of patient history in an evaluation, tracking of signs and symptoms over time, and continuous documentation. Without these items, the patient's true diagnosis may have been missed and ultimately resulted in a ruptured cyst or other sequelae. Additionally, the discussion of all aspects of a condition, including risk during participation, is also highlighted in this case. The athlete and her parents all agreed to her continued participation in basketball when the differential diagnosis was presented. Constant communication and monitoring then became a paramount cornerstone of this athlete-athletic trainer relationship.

A strength of this case is the incorporation, with permission by the patient, of her parents. Allowing the patient to actively contribute to her care plan by informing the people she desired to be involved in her care strengthened the overall care process. I believe one of the reasons this patient had such a successful outcome and could complete her basketball season prior to undergoing surgery was that she was given all of the available information and was able to make an informed decision with her family. Her values and desires were considered every step of the way in consult with other members of the care team.

In reflection, this case, which occurred early in my career, marked the need for general medical knowledge by an athletic trainer. We are often the first health care provider that an athlete will go to with an issue. Sometimes what seems orthopedic in nature at first is actually the manifestation of symptoms of a more advanced underlying medical condition. We need to not only be aware of these conditions and know when to refer, but we need to be comfortable enough in our knowledge to assist as an active participant in the care plan for athletes who develop these "zebra" diagnoses.

TRUST YOUR EDUCATION

Morgan Cooper Bagley PhD, AT, ATC

KEY TERMS

Postconcussion Syndrome | Arnold Chiari Malformation

Concussions have been a popular topic over the last 5 years, but what if it is more than just a concussion? What if you disagree with the diagnosis? Do you know what to do next? This is a story of knowing your patient and doing what is best, even when you disagree with other medical professionals.

TRUE STORY #16

An 18-year-old female soccer goalie went up to catch a penalty kick and was hit in the face with the soccer ball just lateral to the zygomatic bone. The patient did not present with difficulty recalling memories or balance. She complained of a headache and nausea. The patient had a previous history of 4 diagnosed concussions over the past 5 years. The patient was clinically diagnosed with a concussion.

The patient did not return to practice that day and was referred to the team physician for evaluation. He concurred with the diagnosis and 13 days postinjury the athlete stated her symptoms were resolved and was cleared to return to practice by the team physician, but the soccer season was over so she did not return to practice. Eighteen days postconcussion, the patient returned to the athletic trainer complaining of headaches and having difficulty with memory recall. She had gone to a haunted house the night before and that was when her symptoms returned. She was referred to the team physician where he ordered a magnetic resonance imaging (MRI) of her brain. The MRI did not show any brain abnormalities and she was referred to a neurologist.

Almost 2 months postconcussion, the neurologist and team physician cleared her to practice as able, but the athletic trainer objected stating that the patient was still not acting herself and she was still having symptoms. The athletic trainer spoke with the team physician and the team physician agreed and did not allow the patient to return to playing sports.

In February of the following year, the athlete came to see the athletic trainer stating that she was having symptoms including light sensitivity, blurred vision, headaches, sleeplessness, and general fatigue. She was referred to the neurologist who ordered a cervical MRI, a glucose study, a sleep study, and neuropsychological exam. She was referred to a cognitive-neurological doctor. At this point, the athlete and her family decided it was best for her to medically withdraw from school so that she could continue treatment with her physicians and focus on getting healthy.

The cervical MRI revealed a Type I Arnold Chiari malformation. The glucose test results showed hypoglycemia. The sleep study results showed hypersomnia. Following these results, she was referred to a neurology surgeon, a sports dietician, and a cognitive therapist. She was still having all symptoms as listed before and had developed depression due to an inability to improve and being forced to drop out of school.

The following summer, now almost 2 years postinjury, the athlete was scheduled for surgery to correct the Type 1 Arnold Chiari malformation. Following surgery, she continued rehabilitation and seeing a counselor. One year after medically withdrawing, the patient returned to college as a part time student. Her rehabilitation was continued with her school's athletic training department. Fast forward 4 years she is still attending school part time and hopes to graduate this fall, 6 years postinjury. She still has symptoms and may have postconcussion symptoms for the remainder of her life.

REFLECTION

Athletic trainers are taught to be ready for anything. We are well-educated health care professionals and need to have confidence in our abilities. The athletic trainer in this story was told by the neurologist that if the patient had returned to play soccer there was a chance that it could have cost the patient her life. The athletic trainer trusted her educational background and, using evidence-based best practice with concussion management, did not let the athlete return to play.

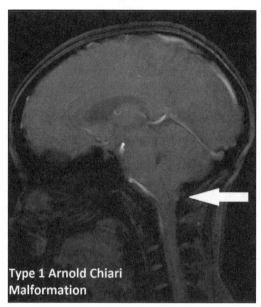

Figure 16-1. Cervical magnetic resonance imaging of a Type I Arnold Chiari malformation.

Bilateral Anterior Cruciate Ligament Tear in a Female Junior Varsity High School Basketball Player

Ryan Johnson, LAT, ATC

Key Terms

Anterior Cruciate Ligament | Medial Collateral Ligament | Patella Subluxation

Working as an athletic trainer in the secondary school setting has its challenges both logistically and physically; however, to me, the most challenging aspect for any athletic trainer is never knowing what injury or illness is going to walk, hobble, or crutch through the door. I think most athletic trainers have that one story that makes their colleagues say, "Wow, I've never seen that in all the years I've worked as an athletic trainer." This is one of those stories that makes you scratch your head and say, "Wow, I never even thought that was possible."

True Story #17

I was working at Holt High School outside of Lansing, Michigan as the only certified athletic trainer on-site. I was covering a junior varsity girl's basketball game on a night that my athletic director said, "Should be a short night," considering the team we were playing only had 6 players and hadn't won a game all season. We've all worked those blowout games that are hard to watch and stay focused, but this was an excruciatingly painful game to watch. The opposing team could barely dribble the ball up the court, let alone come close to scoring a bucket.

So I looked up with a minute left in the first half and my team was winning 42-0 and I thought, well at least we will get a running clock in the second half. At that point I noticed one of my players dived out of bounds under our own basket at the far end of the court. She had tried to save the ball by throwing it between her legs while jumping out of bounds and landed awkwardly, right foot, left foot, then fell to both knees. She was in immediate pain and filled the mostly empty gym with screams of agony.

As I hurried across the court to get to her, my initial thought was she had just landed awkwardly on both of her knees and she probably had a contusion of either or both knees. When I got to her I asked her if was it her knee. She responded, "Yes". I asked which knee was it. She looked at me like I was crazy and said, "Both" with a frantic look in her eyes. Again, I thought, big deal, that supports my original thought of a possible contusion, so I asked her that one decisive question every athletic trainer ask when evaluating a knee. "Did you hear or feel a pop or a snap?" She responded, "Yes, I felt a bunch of pops in both knees."

It was not the response I had anticipated, so I proceeded to perform a Lachman's test on the left knee first, which had some laxity so I compared it to the right knee. The right knee had laxity as well, but it was consistent with the contralateral side. She had tenderness over the medial patellofemoral ligament on both knees and showed signs of discomfort with a patella apprehension test. She also had medial collateral ligament (MCL) tenderness on her right knee and presented with a positive valgus stress test. I checked for a tibial pulse, which was present, and had the coach help me chair carry the athlete to the athletic training room so I could get her on a table and get a better feel for the special test.

By time we got her on the table, edema had set in on both knees and she was guarding too much to get a good end point on her anterior cruciate ligament (ACL) or test the integrity of her meniscus. My prognosis that night was a bilateral patella subluxation in addition to a right MCL sprain. I only had one knee immobilizer at the time (it was a rough year and all of my other immobilizers were in use) so I immobilized her right knee to help give stability to her MCL. When I pulled out a pair of crutches the athlete was not amused, but after some practicing bearing the weight on her left leg she was able to crutch out of my athletic training room.

At this point the game was over. I looked up at the scoreboard to see it was 63-0. My coach was in total disbelief when I gave him the prognosis. Neither of us understood why the athlete was trying to save the ball from going out of bounds in a game where the outcome was all but decided. I will note that my coach did take all the starters out at the start of the second half and intentionally tried to let the other team score. Still, they couldn't make a basket.

I was able to get the athlete an appointment to see our orthopedic surgeon at Michigan State University sports medicine department within a day or 2. The doctor came to a similar conclusion that she had subluxed both patellas and had an grade 2 MCL sprain on the right side. He wrote her a script for physical therapy. I was a little anxious when he initially didn't order the magnetic resonance imaging to check the integrity of her ACL on both knees, but he felt the laxity was equal bilaterally and decided to try physical therapy for 3 weeks to help with the edema and pain tolerance.

After 3 weeks, she wasn't responding well to physical therapy so when she followed up with the orthopedic surgeon he ordered an MRI on her right knee first. The imaging showed she had a classic triad (ACL, MCL, medial meniscus tear) on her right knee, which surprised the doctor so he ordered an magnetic resonance imaging on her left knee just to make sure. When the results came back she had also torn her ACL in her left knee.

So, my athlete had a triad and patella subluxation in her right knee, and a complete ACL tear with a patella subluxation in her left knee, all of which happened via a single mechanism in a junior varsity girl's basketball game that our team won 63-0. It serves as a lesson, you never know what injury will come knocking at your door. Whether you team is up 63-0 or down 63-0, injuries have no bias.

The orthopedic surgeon eventually repaired her left ACL first and let her recover for 4 weeks before repairing her right ACL and medial meniscus. She would go on to have multiple scopes in her right knee to debride the excess scar tissue but was eventually able to return to contact sports after 12 months of rehabilitation.

REFLECTION

Looking back on that night, I never even considered the possibility that this athlete could have torn both ACLs only because I had never heard of this much bilateral trauma in athletics. After we received the MRI results, I searched through case studies and could only find bilateral ACL tears in patients in the military and automobile accidents. In this day and age, ACL tears are almost always in the forefront of people's mind when an athlete go down holding their knee; however, a bilateral ACL tear seems almost unimaginable and very unlikely to occur in athletics. As athletic trainers, we are taught to compare the integrity of a ligament or joint to the contralateral side; however, our ability to effectively evaluate an athlete with a bilateral ailment is compromised without the assistance of additional imaging.

This is by far the most unique case that I have ever treated as an athletic trainer and will always remember this athlete for her hard work and determination to return to athletics. Since that day I have made it a point to emphasize attentiveness when providing coverage, no matter what level of athletics or the score or outcome of those events.

Domain III

Immediate and Emergency Care

CERVICAL SPINE MANAGEMENT
LUCK MEETS PREPARATION

Robert J. Casmus, MS, ATC

KEY TERMS

Concussion | Cervical | Emergency Action Plan | Retrolisthesis | Stabilization

---

Cervical spine injuries in football can be catastrophic and decision making should be to err on the side of caution. Successful management truly involves a team effort with everyone working together towards the same goal of putting the patient's best interest first. Rehearsing both the emergency action plan and spine boarding procedures are a must. Coordinating with emergency response personnel is crucial for transitioning the athlete from the field to the emergency room. Good communication is required for a successful outcome.

grammar

TRUE STORY #18

I remember looking at the practice clock and thinking that in about 15 to 20 seconds this Saturday morning football practice will end (at noon) and in another 2 hours I will be on the golf course with 2 friends of mine. Both of my golfing pals by the way are physicians and brothers. One is a dentist/maxilla-facial surgeon and the other happens to be a neurosurgeon. This was the last true contact practice of the preseason as freshmen orientation would start later in the day and the fall semester classes would begin on Wednesday. The upperclassmen would have the rest of the day free and the team would not practice again until tomorrow evening. From tomorrow forward, all football practices would occur just once a day with minimal contact as game week was just around the corner. That practice clock couldn't count down fast enough.

With about 10 seconds to go, the last play of the day started. A pass was thrown to a receiver and 2 defensive backs were breaking on the ball. These 2 defensive backs were roommates and best friends. The receiver turned the wrong way on the pass

Gorse KM, Feld F, Blanc RO, eds.
True Stories From the Athletic Training Room (pp 61-85).
© 2018 SLACK Incorporated.

route, tripped and fell, and collided with both defenders who also fell to the ground. This did not look good. I started taking those baby-steps from the sidelines towards them hoping that they would just pop up off the ground. The receiver got up and ran towards his huddle. The one defensive back laid face-up and did not move while the other rolled up, rubbed his thigh and then stood up. Now I began the athletic trainer "jog-run" to the athlete in question who still was not moving.

When I got to the athlete, he was conscious and alert. I asked Billy (not his real name) what happened and what was going on. He related that his neck and left hand really hurt. In my mind, I was thinking, "Ok, here we go—got to think the worst and hope I am wrong!" I stabilized his head and went through all the steps for on-field cervical spine evaluation. He could move his feet and bend his knees on his own. He could flex his elbows and move his wrists bilaterally. Billy could wiggle his fingers on this right hand but not all of them on his left because it hurt too much. I had the senior athletic training student go through the sensory evaluation of his lower extremity and upper extremity which was fully intact. His grip strength was reported to be good on the right but weak on the left. With one hand, I gently palpated what I could of his neck and he related that this too was painful. Fortunately there was no gross spasm or deformity.

Following this, I encouraged Billy not to move his head or neck but to stay still. Per the quickie concussion evaluation, he was alert and oriented to time, person, place, and location. He had full recall of the event and remembered diving for the ball and he believed he had hit his head on his teammate's thigh. He did not recall blacking out or having heard a pop or snap. His chief complaint was severe neck pain and his left hand hurt. He did not report any burning, numbness or tingling to any of his extremities other than the pain in his left hand. A pulse oximeter was applied to the right index finger so I could check his vital signs. The vital signs I believed would be good based on the on-going oral communication that I was having with this fully-conscious and alert athlete. No surprise that his vital signs taken were within normal limits.

At this moment, I had basically all the information I could gather per an initial on-field cervical spine evaluation. Now was the time to make the critical decision. I knew this athlete was not a whiner, crier, or complainer. He is a pretty tough kid and not a "frequent flyer" in the athletic training room. I didn't believe he was exaggerating his cervical pain and he clearly had left hand pain and weak grip strength. His mechanism of injury matched that of potential cervical spine trauma. My gut feeling was that it is OK and smart to play it safe. We activated the emergency action plan and it ran smooth to a point. Good news was that athletic training students knew during the evaluation process to bring over our emergency equipment to have handy and alongside. They were ready with the oxygen tank, suction, automated external defibrillator, spine board and cervical collars. They even brought the notebook that had the emergency contact information for the athletes. I was very proud of them for being on-top of their game. One put a cell phone next to my face so I could contact and speak with the 911 dispatcher and request emergency assistance. A stroke of luck was that my golfing buddy was a neurosurgeon. Once emergency medical services arrived, I might have chance to contact him directly and get him involved with this potential cervical spine case.

Up until this point, everything was sailing along smoothly. The athlete was calm and compliant. The coaches and athletic training students were doing the right thing and being supportive. Billy's face mask came off without any issues using the portable drill and a cervical collar was applied. Our campus security office was also notified, and they were going to guide the ambulance to the practice field. Per local town protocol, the fire department first responders will arrive ahead of the paramedics and/or emergency medical technicians for trauma calls. Another stroke of fortune is that the fire department is literally 2 blocks from campus. The firemen use our weight room and track for their fitness and exercise programs which are next to our football practice field, so they knew where to go from the start. Having certified adult first responders assist with placing a pretty good sized individual onto a spine board is, in my opinion, quite beneficial. We rehearsed cervical spine protocol with the athletic training students 2 days prior to the football team's arrival for preseason. In reality, not all athletic training students have the same strength per moving an injured athlete onto a spine board or even helping someone up off the ground. This is an example of a situation that having good strength is crucial. Another case where luck meets preparation is that in early July, I did my annual guest speaker session with the county EMS and fire personnel on the recommended protocol for taking care of the on-field football player with potential cervical spine injury.

Within minutes of notifying EMS via 911, the firemen first responders arrived on the scene. The first words out of the lead responder's mouth were that the football helmet had to come off right away. I responded that it is not the proper procedure for handling a potential cervical spine injured football player. In my mind I thought, is this guy crazy or what? What did I just teach and go over with you folks last month? I knew this was not the place and nor the time to have an argument. In a rather stern and direct manner, I said to the first responders, this is how we are going to manage this athlete and we are going to maintain his cervical spine stabilization with his equipment on. We are going to lift and slide him onto the spine board per my commands. They responded that the local protocol directs them to log roll cervical spine patients. My response was that on this campus, my physician protocol will direct our actions and we will do a lift and slide as we have the necessary helpers. I added that since the patient is face-up, we will greatly limit any cervical motion using the lift and slide. Again, this was spoken in a stern but confident manner. Fortunately, the firemen first responders agreed to my directives and the athlete was transferred accordingly to the spine board with me still maintaining cervical spine stabilization.

The paramedic and EMT soon arrived with the ambulance just after we spine boarded Billy. They completed their assessment and had no issues with the football equipment being kept on the athlete patient. The paramedic and I both recognized each other from my presentation in July so I believe that helped avoid any further conflicts regarding football equipment removal. The patient, while spine boarded and collared, was placed on the stretcher and then loaded into the ambulance as I still maintained cervical spine stabilization. At this point, I was told by the EMS personnel that I had to remove my hands and could not ride in the back but was welcome to ride in the passenger seat to the hospital. They explained that only county EMS personnel are only permitted in the back of the ambulance where patient care is provided. I personally would have liked to continue maintaining cervical spine stabilization on the way to the hospital which is located literally a mile and a half from campus. Rather than create a scene and explain to the paramedics that I was currently a certified EMT, a certified athletic trainer, and that I was probably more than qualified to ride in the back, I relinquished cervical spine stabilization. I knew the athlete was stable and not in acute life-threatening distress. Now would be my chance to contact my neurosurgeon friend via cell phone for his input and assistance as Billy was being transported to the hospital. While in route, I also notified our school president, vice president for athletics, and the director of athletics of this potential catastrophic injury. On a small college campus, rumors can run wild and I wanted them to hear direct information from me. I chose to delay calling Billy's grandmother (his guardian) until I knew for sure what his true condition was and what would be diagnosed in the emergency room. My protocol has been not to call and worry or upset parents until I had definitive information to provide them.

My next concern was how the emergency department personnel would deal with this athlete, his cumbersome equipment and my persistence to see that he was managed appropriately. Hospital personnel have never been receptive to my offer to provide training or a lecture in managing an athlete with a cervical spine injury and football equipment issues. The stars and planets must have been aligned in the right place as the attending emergency room physician asked who I was and allowed me to offer advice and suggestions per this situation. I am sure that my neurosurgeon friend made a phone call as well with the suggestion to use my knowledge and skills. After the emergency physician did her evaluation, it was discovered that Billy had a dislocated left fourth digit at the proximal interphalangeal joint. This greatly explained his left hand pain and weak grip strength. The dislocated joint was reduced but Billy still had the mechanism of injury for a cervical spine injury and he still had the persistent cervical pain that never improved or diminished. My advice was to allow me to don the lead vest and have a portable X-ray take initial views of the cervical spine with the football equipment in place. I told the doctor this would at least give you a rough idea if there is any apparent boney fracture or dislocation. I would pull and distract his arms in such a way that maybe cervical vertebrae 6 and/or 7 could be viewed. If these X-rays were negative, the football equipment could be removed and then either an magnetic resonance imaging (MRI) or computerized tomography (CT) scan could be ordered for further testing. Alternatively, if there was any fracture at least she would know what might be underlying and could consult with the neurosurgeon on call. I did not relate that I had already spoken to my neurosurgeon friend as I did not want to cause any undue friction with the case as he was not officially on-call. These steps were agreed to after taking the initial X-rays and then proceeding forwards pending the results.

Initial plain view X-rays showed something suspicious to the ER physician at cervical level 5 and 6, but the films were not clear enough due to the football equipment. My advice at this time was to remove the equipment—meaning the helmet and shoulder pads simultaneously. The patient was alert, conscious, and stable per vital signs. Billy had full motor and sensory response to the upper and lower extremities. The ER physician agreed and with the help of 4 nurses we successfully removed the football equipment. The football jersey and shoulder pad straps were cut. The cheek pads were pried out and the chin strap was cut as the physician maintained cervical spine traction. The helmet was removed and the shoulder pads slid out from under the athlete. I have to applaud these individuals as this was their first time doing this procedure and they did spectacular. The athlete who was still wearing a cervical collar and still on the spine board was transferred to the CT scan unit.

The CT scan report was not a good one as Billy had a teardrop fracture at C5. There was also retrolisthesis of C5 and C6 with abnormal disc height loss and mild angulation across the level of the disc. The interspinsous space was abnormally enlarged along with abnormal diastases of the C5 and C6 facets. There was direct compression of the ventral spinal cord by the posterior inferior margin of C5 as well as a large amount of ruptured disc material into the spinal canal. Additionally, the spinal canal was narrowed to 5 mm in the anterior-posterior dimension.

It was recommended by the neurosurgeon in consult with the attending emergency room physician to transport this athlete to a level one trauma center. Our local hospital did not have the required surgical staffing and equipment to handle this complicated case that required surgical intervention. Billy was then prepared to be transferred to the level one trauma center which was located about 35 miles away from campus. At this time, I notified Billy's grandmother and explained the situation and what was being done for his care. I held the phone to Billy's mouth so he could talk with her in order to alleviate any high level distress she may undergo. My next step was to notify our head football coach and campus personnel of the situation and the decisions being made. I noted that I would also be accompanying this athlete to the level one trauma center. I also recommended that we should all meet at the trauma center to offer support to Billy and his family.

As I followed the transporting ambulance taking Billy to the trauma center, I remembered that one of our former team physicians from 10 years earlier was now the head of orthopedics and sports medicine at the trauma. I called him on his cell phone and asked if he could look in on the case and help keep me updated as I did not think the attending physicians and surgeons would allow me access to Billy once he got to the trauma center. He said he would make some calls on my behalf and do what he could but this was not his department and even his influence may not be strong enough to get the assistance I requested. Whatever phone call he made had me dealt an ace and a 10 for blackjack! The trauma center knew I was coming and the hospital personnel permitted me full access to Billy. The physicians and surgeons on Billy's trauma team were supportive and informative. The sports medicine department residents even came by and checked in on Billy and me and collaborated with the trauma team. The trauma team, following an additional MRI of the cervical spine, decided to operate the next day to stabilize Billy's cervical spine fracture and repair the herniated discs. He was slid off the spine board onto a bed and kept in his cervical collar. Family members soon arrived and so did our head campus administrators and head football coach. I left Billy's side around midnight to go home for some sleep as I would be back the next day.

Billy had a successful outcome per his surgical repair. He walked out of the hospital 5 days later and returned to classes 7 days post-trauma. The trauma team physicians told us both that normally patients with his condition coming into the trauma center don't always have as good an outcome as he did. Billy no longer played football but he got to walk across the stage at graduation 2 years later and pick up his diploma.

REFLECTION

This catastrophic event had a great outcome, and I caught quite a few lucky breaks. Fortunately, I practiced and rehearsed spine boarding and reviewed the emergency action plan with the students prior to preseason football. I am most grateful for their bringing their "A-game" to football practice that day. Mostly, I appreciate Billy for landing face-up and having stable vital signs. Communication is key and even with the best of preparation, one has to be ready for the worst. It is important to go through the evaluation and diagnostic steps for the catastrophic injured athlete without cutting corners or rushing through it. My instinct was to play it safe and if I looked like a fool calling 911/EMS for what could have been just a neck strain, I could still sleep well at night. A good decision was made and the outcome was equally as good. Every chance I get to speak or volunteer to speak to local EMS personnel, I jump at the chance. Most of them know who I am and know that I am a health care professional with the education and training to handle such emergencies as a football player with potential cervical injury. It is important to be in control of the situation when those around you are inexperienced or not up-to-date on proper emergency procedures such as the football equipped athlete. A team effort is needed to do what is in the athlete's best interest and not create a scene or a "territorial battle." Communication, again, was a key factor in creating a positive outcome. Experience has taught me to make connections and network with the various medical providers in my town as one never knows when those resources are going to be needed or utilized. I truly appreciate the friendships that I have made with our various local physician specialists. One of my follow-up steps was to write and thank the emergency room physician for her support and care for Billy. I even promoted her professionalism towards me and her top-notch emergency care for Billy with the hospital CEO. Lastly, I need to keep in mind for the future that whoever is delegated to evaluate and/or palpate the extremities regarding motor and sensor response needs to note whether or not all finger joints are intact without defect or deformity. A finger dislocation—even though a minor and somewhat unimportant issue in the final outcome of this case—did give us false-positive grip strength response. I do believe that, if that was the worst mistake I made with Billy's case, then I did pretty well overall.

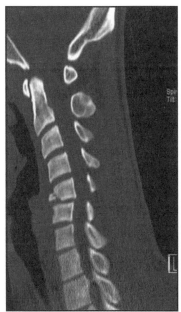

Figure 18-1. Computerized tomography scan image showing C5 fracture with retrolisthesis and narrowing of spinal canal.

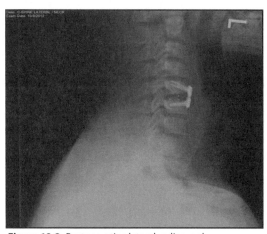

Figure 18-2. Postoperative lateral radiograph.

Preparing for "That Moment"

Kyle Johnston, MS, ATC, LAT, Blake LeBlanc, PT, DPT, ATC, LAT, and Sam Zuege, MS, ATC, LAT

Key Terms

Emergency Action Plan | Injury Communication | Postinjury Pearls of Wisdom

No matter what point you are at in your career, we've all heard about having your emergency action plan (EAP). We read them, post them, discuss them, and hopefully have rehearsed them to some degree. Admittedly, throughout my career, the main parts of this plan I would concern myself with were the entry points for the ambulance or facility address. In one of my first few years as a head athletic trainer, the importance of having an EAP, the depth in which you discuss it with your staff and how to deal with postcatastrophic injury management was no more apparent than on October 22, 2011.

True Story #19

It's Friday night at Papa John's Cardinal Stadium on October 22, 2011 and we are playing against conference leader, Rutgers University. Our football team was feeling the pressure to get our first conference win of the season with a national audience watching on ESPN. Although the temperature in "The Oven" was rising fast, our sports medicine staff went through our normal gameday procedures.

Our typical pregame routine is no different than anywhere else, including a hospitable welcome to our visiting team's medical staff. This is our opportunity to network, catch up with colleagues, and most importantly discuss our EAP which includes the locations of the ambulance, radiology, hospital location, and spine boarding protocols. This pregame meeting, however, was different than many of the others. A year earlier, Rutgers and their staff had a cervical spine injury that left their student athlete a quadriplegic. We were interested in the health of the student athlete, as well as the handling of the tragic situation. As I walked away from our pregame meeting to head back to the locker room, I subconsciously asked myself, "Are we truly ready to handle a catastrophic injury?"

I was fortunate in my years as an undergraduate and graduate student to have supervisors who routinely reviewed our EAPs and practiced spine boarding. In my first year as the head athletic trainer, my staff and I decided to take our EAP a step further and bring our game day ambulance crew to our facility during the summer to discuss our plans and rehearse several different injury scenarios. We felt it was imperative for everyone to be comfortable with the various techniques used for splinting, spine boarding, transportation, and most importantly, to work through individual roles. We rehearsed everything from retrieving the emergency equipment to loading a victim into the ambulance. During our practice sessions, we recognized that there were several changes to our process we needed to modify. One adjustment related to collecting information during our initial subjective assessments with suspected head and neck injuries. Instead of asking "yes/no" questions, we felt that it was better to ask questions that would make the student athlete cognitively think about how they would answer. Rather than ask the victim, "Do you have a headache?" we asked, "How bad is your headache?" Through our experiences we have come to understand that student athletes, especially in game situations, will likely give you the answer they think they need to give to stay in a game. This subtle change proved to be crucial in the scenario we faced on October 22, 2011.

The first quarter atmosphere was as electric as expected and we had the lead heading into the second quarter. On the first play of the second quarter, all of the air was sucked out of the stadium and all eyes turned their attention to our sports medicine staff. A Rutgers receiver caught a pass down field and our defensive back came up to make the tackle near our sideline. Our cornerback ducked his head to dive at the opposing player's legs to make the tackle. As he made contact, he fell to his back in a "fenced" position. I immediately went to stabilize our player's head and neck, assuming at the minimum we would be dealing with a concussion. I was joined on the field by our head team orthopedic physician and assistant athletic trainer. When we first arrived to our player, he was unconscious but had normal breathing. Within the first 5 to 10 seconds he slowly regained consciousness, and we began our initial assessment. He answered all the cognitive questions we were putting him through appropriately. As we asked him these questions, he began moving his legs and arms. While still maintaining cervical spine stabilization, we asked him, "How bad is the pain in your neck?" His response, "I don't really have pain, just a little bit of a cramp in my trap." This was not a huge red flag, but it was enough to make our sports medicine staff on the field pause for a few seconds. Thinking back to our EAP training, one of the things we emphasized was to take our time to make good, sound, rational decisions in the management of our student athletes. Based on the angle at which we saw his head-on contact and the fact that he had at least a subtle upper extremity symptom, we made the decision to activate our EAP to rule out cervical injury.

We executed our protocol and he was loaded into the ambulance and sent to our downtown hospital for imaging for what we deemed "precautionary reasons." Before leaving in the ambulance, I told him that we would call his mother to let her know that he was doing fine. He acknowledged this and told me to tell her that "he would be fine." He knew she was watching on TV at home in Texas and would be anxiously awaiting the news. As part of our EAP, while the athlete was being carted off the field, an assistant retrieved his emergency contact information out of the binder that we keep for all our players in our sideline emergency bag. This allowed us to immediately call his mother from the sideline after securing him in the ambulance to let her know he was responsive and was moving all extremities. We explained that we wanted to take every precaution necessary to rule out any further orthopedic injuries due to the hit. I told her that if anything changed with his medical status we would notify her immediately, but he would be undergoing several tests. She understood and was appreciative of the call.

After hanging up the phone with his mother, like most athletic trainers, I reflected on our processes and started critiquing a few of the small things that I noticed during the management of our student athlete. Thankfully, I felt the overall process of spine boarding our supine athlete went as smooth as possible. Everyone was calm and stayed within their assigned role. I've been told sometimes perception can be reality. I felt with a national audience, the professionalism and organization with which our EAP was handled reflected the amount of work and preparation we had put in as a staff.

About 20 to 30 minutes later, I received a call from Assistant Athletic Trainer, Sam Zuege, who traveled in the ambulance to the hospital with the student athlete. He asked me to go to a place in a stadium where I could talk privately. After making my way to a secured location, he gave me the news that none of us expected. Our student athlete had suffered a C4 vertebral fracture. The doctors at the hospital indicated the fracture was millimeters away from damaging the spinal cord. He continued to have feeling and control in all extremities; however, the emergency room doctors said that a spine specialist would need to get involved for consultation to ensure appropriate acute management of this serious injury.

Everything up to this phone call was something our staff had prepared for in our EAP. All the events that transpired over the next several hours are things that we never discussed or learned how to manage from a textbook. What do we do with this information? What is the next step? How and when is the appropriate time to communicate the information and plan with the parties involved? Who are the parties that need to be involved?

Some of the best advice that many of us on staff have received from our mentors is to work slowly and methodically through any stressful situation. With this in mind, Sam and I decided that he would handle the management of the student athlete at the hospital and ensure that only select individuals knew the initial findings. To help with this, we had the student athlete registered to the intensive care unit under an alias, allowing only permitted individuals to enter his room. He would continue to update me on subsequent images the student athlete was going to undergo to further give a more detailed diagnosis. Additionally, we decided an athletics staff member would stay with him at all times until his mother was able to travel to Louisville, Kentucky.

On my end, I was going to communicate the information with our Head Team Orthopedic Physician, Dr. Raymond Shea. He would begin contacting the appropriate specialists who would need to be involved with the potential surgical care of this case. Before going back to the game field to discuss the situation with Dr. Shea,

I took several minutes to process the situation and map out a game plan. The game plan included appropriate dissemination of information to doctors, his family, staff, administration, coaches, and his teammates.

Upon returning to the field, I relayed the initial radiographic results with the rest of our staff and told them to keep the information confidential as we were still gathering information. I then discussed with Dr. Shea what Sam had relayed from the hospital and we planned the next steps. We both agreed it would be best to collect as much information as possible to devise a concrete care plan before contacting his family so we could be prepared to answer any questions. In the meantime, we did not want to spread any information to coaches or fellow teammates to avoid any in-game distractions or inaccurate information being leaked.

Around the beginning of the fourth quarter, we had all the medical details finalized. Fusion of C3 through C5 was recommended and the specialist involved said that surgical intervention could wait until his mother arrived to town. Our next immediate call went to our administration which included our athletic director and associate athletic director of compliance. We felt it was necessary to get administration involved before talking to his family so we could get clearance and approval to assist in travel and lodging accommodations. We knew his mother's top priority was to be with her son, especially once she received the official diagnosis. After gaining clearance from our compliance officer, I went inside to call his mother on a land line to talk in a quiet place and ensure there were no reception issues on our end. I decided it was important for our team chaplain to accompany me for this call, having already established relationships, through previous instances, we knew the family was grounded in their faith.

The next person to update was the head coach, and subsequently, the rest of our coaching staff, and most importantly, his teammates. As mentioned previously, we did not want this injury to be a distraction to the outcome of the game. We knew the significance of the injury would take the coaches time to digest before determining the best way to inform his teammates. I waited until about 3 minutes to go in the game before giving our head coach the diagnosis and tentative plans.

Immediately following the game, we accessed the student athlete's medical file to verify that he had signed the release waiver giving us permission to release medical information to the news media. After addressing the team in the locker room, the head coach, myself and the assistant sports information director discussed how we would handle the news media. We felt it was best to stick with our typical protocol of the head coach being the only person who would discuss the student athlete's condition. I advised coach that each time he addressed the media over the next several days that he read a prepared statement just giving basic information and to not field questions on specifics. Considering each injury that requires surgery can have complications, we agreed it was best to not elaborate on any prognosis or predictions until his surgery was complete and he was getting discharged from the hospital. The initial statement read: "(Name omitted) suffered a cervical fracture tonight during the second quarter. He was transported to a local hospital for evaluation and medical care. He will remain in the hospital until a surgical procedure is performed to stabilize his injury. He continues to maintain good feeling and movement in all extremities. We will provide another update during the Monday press conference."

On Monday, the prepared statement read: "(Name omitted) will have a surgical procedure done today at Jewish Hospital by Dr. (Name omitted). The surgery will be done to help stabilize his cervical fracture. (Name omitted) continues to maintain good feeling and movement in all his extremities."

The day after the game, our sports medicine staff and doctors reviewed the whole scenario. We reviewed TV coverage of the game as well as other still pictures to help us assess how the injury management looked. Anytime we initiate our EAP, we meet to evaluate our actions so we can continue to improve our procedures. We were fortunate in the assessment of this injury management because we had media resources to utilize.

The student athlete had successful surgery to fuse C3 through C5. In the days and months that ensued we followed the physician's rehabilitation plan closely. We also incorporated psychological support from the various resources we have on our campus to help the student athlete cope with the realization that his football career was over. However, one of the most influential moments in his postinjury management was a phone call he received while still in the hospital. The young man from Rutgers University, who just one year earlier suffered a cervical spine injury which left him with paralysis, placed a call to our student athlete. This conversation left a huge impression on our individual. He realized that he was lucky and he could use his situation to influence people just as his counterpart was doing from Rutgers.

As our student athlete moved through his postsurgical rehabilitation, he found ways to become a major influence not only in our program, but also with the children in the Louisville community. His message and mission was to convey how important an education is. Over the ensuing months, he followed his own words and obtained his college degree. In April of 2012, he received the Inspiration Award at our annual athletic department awards ceremony. It was a joy for our staff to watch him walk across the stage with a smile on his face as he received this recognition.

REFLECTION

Discussing, rehearsing and evaluating your EAP is extremely important. Understanding that you are practicing for not "if" but "when" something catastrophic will occur in your career. Everyone involved should have a deep understanding of their roles and responsibilities, hopefully providing a strong foundation and blueprint for having successful outcomes in injury management. Your actions immediately following a catastrophic event can also greatly affect the overall outcome. In the heat of the moment, take your time and rationalize what is best for the student athlete and everyone else that may be involved.

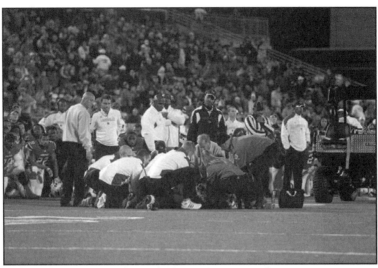

Figure 19-1. Photograph of an on-field emergency action plan.

THE EYES HAVE IT

Francis Feld, DNP, CRNA, LAT, ATC, NRP

KEY TERMS

Spinal Injury | EAP | Life-changing Events

During the course of our lives, we all experience events that are so compelling we often refer to them as life changing. Some of these events are personal such as getting married, having a child, getting divorced, or experiencing the death of a loved one. Other events are on a professional level and may cause us to choose or leave a career, change jobs, or significantly alter the way we practice. These events are so profound, that we think of them on a daily basis and although over time the frequency may wane, it never disappears.

My professional career has had 2 life-changing events and although I never thought they were connected, I now see that the first ultimately led to the second. The process took 32 years, but I am comfortable with the result.

TRUE STORY #20

Upon graduation from the University of Pittsburgh (Pitt) in April of 1976, I had no clear idea of where my professional career was headed. I had spent 4 years as a student athletic trainer at Pitt and completed the internship route to certification with extensive football experience. I returned home about 60 miles north of Pittsburgh and went to work for a local bus company driving charters into Pittsburgh and volunteering at the local fire department. I wanted to be an athletic trainer and had registered to take the National Athletic Trainers' Association exam in August, but didn't have any other plans. Briefly, I looked into getting a commission in the U.S. Marine Corps but my parents; both Navy veterans of World War II nixed that idea quickly.

Late in the summer, Pitt Head Athletic Trainer, Tim Karin, called me about a high school 30 miles from me that was looking to hire an athletic trainer. The process moved quickly and I was soon interviewing with the school board at Center High

School in Beaver County. I was 22 and quite overwhelmed but now I was the first full-time athletic trainer at a high school in the area. The next 2 years were a pleasant work experience and I quickly adapted to the tasks required because of strong support from a great team physician, a principal that was interactive, and a football coach that quickly adapted to a new staff member. I thought I was ready for anything.

In late spring 1978, Pitt came calling and I returned to the university as the assistant football athletic trainer. Center High School tried to keep me, but I had to answer the siren call of a bigger stadium. I sometimes wonder what might have happened if I had stayed at Center High School since the state pension plan is very robust and I would have been able to retire after 30 years with a sizable pension. Monday morning quarterbacking is a great thing but it really has no value.

Starting at Pitt in May, I dove into my work and jumped at all the opportunities that came up. That summer, the local chapter of a charitable organization decided to hold an all-star football game with players from Western Pennsylvania playing. An athletic trainer from a local small college and myself were the athletic trainers for the event and we held practices at Pitt stadium. The week of joint practices went well and I got to meet a lot of great players and high school coaches. The game was held at a local high school that had a turf field (something quite rare then) on Friday, July 21, 1978. A defensive back from my team came up to make a tackle, ducked his head, made the tackle, and hit the ground hard. He didn't get up. I quickly ran to his side and asked what was wrong. He looked at me and said, "Fran, I can't move my legs." The look of stark terror in his eyes has stayed with me to this day. Many of the subsequent events have faded from memory but that look in his eyes haunt me to this day.

Mark, the other athletic trainer, quickly recognized the severity of the injury and was at my side within seconds. We called emergency medical services (EMS) onto the field, immobilized him, and he was transported to a local hospital. The game continued with little enthusiasm and I couldn't tell you who won. I doubt anybody else can tell you either. Mark and I heard the player had been transferred to a larger hospital in Pittsburgh so we both went to the emergency room. We got little information until finally in the early hours of July 22, we were told he was being transferred to yet another hospital in the city for emergency surgery. We left without seeing Jeff.

It soon became apparent that the charitable organization did not have adequate insurance to cover a catastrophic event such as this and talk of lawsuit came up quickly. I never saw Jeff or his family again and when the lawsuit was finally filed, one of the accusations was failure to provide adequate medical care on the field. That shocked me but I was assured that it was only a legal tactic and neither Mark nor I was named in the suit. I never heard of the disposition and I was never deposed so I presume it was settled out of court. Many of the events from that night soon faded although I only had to close my eyes and think of Jeff to see that look of terror in his eyes.

Throughout my time at Pitt, I became increasingly interested in medical issues and read as much as I could find, which, considering this was before the internet, it wasn't always easy. When going to the operating room with our team orthopedic surgeon, I was interested in the surgery but also what was happening at the head of the table where the nurse anesthetist sat. Many were very nice and explained what they were doing although some were pretty nasty and chased me away. My interest was peaked although I didn't realize it at the time.

After 8 years at Pitt, the Pittsburgh Steelers called and I was soon working on the other side of the city at Three Rivers Stadium. Life was different in the National Football League as compared to college and I found myself working at least 30 hours less each week. This gave me time in the evening to take an emergency medical technician and paramedic class, which solved my desire for more medical education and working with my local EMS agency gave me field experience. Throughout all of this, the look in Jeff's eyes never went away although I thought about him less often.

The siren call of the big stadiums had given way to the real siren of an ambulance. Since I was vested in the National Football League pension plan, it seemed like a good time to change careers. Paramedics didn't make much at that time and neither did athletic trainers for that matter. Nursing held the promise of a good job, decent pay, and the ability to move around and not get bored. Boredom was what had made me think of leaving athletic training because routine athletic injuries were just too mundane for me and I craved the excitement of emergency and critical care.

The process moved quickly and I earned a Bachelors of Science in nursing, worked as an registered nurse in an intensive care unit and emergency department to gain experience and graduated with an Masters of Science in nurse anesthesia within 5 years. My first job was at the level one trauma and burn center where I had sat in the ED waiting to hear word about Jeff so many years before. After 16 years specializing in cardiac, neurological, and trauma anesthesia, I moved to a large community hospital closer to home where I specialize in thoracic and esophageal surgery. Difficult cases with very sick patients, but the eyes are still with me.

It is probably safe to say that I am the only person in the country that has taken care of a spine injured football player as an athletic trainer on the field, as a paramedic transporting a player to the hospital, as an RN in the ED where I had to remove the equipment because nobody else knew how, and as a nurse anesthetist where I had to intubate and manage the anesthetic for a player undergoing spinal fusion. In each and every case, Jeff was there and his eyes made me think hard and concentrate on doing my job at the highest level. On September 29, 2013, Jeff was involved in a serious motor vehicle crash and both Jeff and his father were seriously injured. Jeff never left the hospital and succumbed to his injuries in January 2014. He was 54 years old.

It has occurred to me on several occasions that I should have reached out to Jeff and his family over the years, but I really did not know what I would have said. I only knew Jeff for one week before he was injured and rendered a quadriplegic so there wasn't a strong relationship. Still, the look in his eyes has stayed with me over the decades and eventually made me change my career path away from athletic training, although I still maintain my license. It made me realize there was more to health care than orthopedics and sports injuries and I was fortunate enough to be able to pursue and succeed in other areas. One constant in the process has been the look of terror in Jeff's eyes. That has not gone away and I hope it never does because it keeps me humble and aware that no matter how tough my day is going, I always realize that somebody else is having a tougher day and life.

This was never more apparent than when I experienced the second life-changing event in 2010. My federal disaster medical team was deployed by the Department of Health and Human Services to Haiti shortly after the devastating earthquake destroyed the island. I spent 9 days administering anesthesia in a field surgical hospital and worked on average 18 hours per day. One case in particular reminded me of how lucky I am and how hard it is to remain humble. A young man was carried into the operating tent on a stretcher with a lower leg fracture. He had a backpack on his belly and when the stretcher was placed on the operating framework, the backpack fell to the ground. He immediately lunged for it and almost upended the entire table. We caught him before he hit the ground and got the stretcher secured. I placed the backpack on his belly and put his hand on it while I put him to sleep. It occurred to me that everything in the world this young man owned was in that backpack. When the surgery was done, I woke him up but made sure that the backpack was still on his belly and both hands were on it. The eyes had brought me to this place and were with me again.

REFLECTION

Much has changed over the years and some things you think are constant turn out to be fleeting. Both Pitt and Three Rivers Stadiums have been torn down and Center High School merged with Monaca High and now forms Central Valley School District. Many of the fine coaches, athletic trainers, and players I worked with over the years have passed away. And yet it is amazing how one part of a catastrophic injury so many years ago can stay with you and be readily called to mind. The event wasn't the only reason I changed careers, but it was certainly one of them. Since then, I have cared for many patients with very serious injuries; some of them survived while others did not. None affected me as much as Jeff did. I mentioned that Monday morning quarterbacking has no value and while I would not change anything I did on the field that day in July 1978, I do wish I had made an effort to visit Jeff and his family after the injury. Perhaps that is one of the reasons why the look in his eyes has stayed with me to this day. Haunting to be sure, but they have kept me focused and I hope humble.

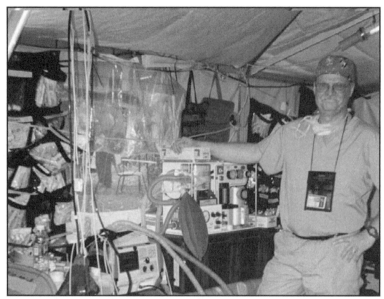

Figure 20-1. Photograph of Dr. Francis Feld in the Haiti operating room.

Heat-Related Illness, Emergency Medicine

Ryan McGovern, MS, LAT, ATC

Key Terms

Heat-related Illness | Emergency Medicine

I was about to start working as a graduate assistant athletic trainer for a collegiate football team in Georgia. I arrived at the beginning of June and immediately began working the annual football camps that were held at the university. The first day of camp was located on 2 artificial turf fields and the temperature was forecast in the low 100s. Not only was it going to be hot, but the humidity made it feel as if you were breathing through a straw. I don't remember much from that day, but I do recollect almost passing out and being escorted inside due to my inability to function in the oppressive heat. While I was no longer an athlete, I considered myself to have been in good enough shape with proper hydration habits. It didn't matter. To this day I am still ridiculed by my former coworkers about that incident. I can't say I blame them; I was just standing there watching.

True Story #21

While that introduction has practically nothing to do with my story, for those who have never worked in the south it sets up the reality of what the encompassing summer had in store. As the 2 weeks of camp progressed, I began to become accustomed to the heat. I dare say that I was actually enjoying the constant sunshine despite the heat and humidity. That was until the last day of camp arrived. This camp was for high school student athletes and was viewed as a large recruiting opportunity for our university. If you have never worked collegiate football, we take these recruiting events very seriously. It is a way to not only have full access to recruits, but it allows student athletes and their families to become acquainted with the coaching staff, support staff, and facilities. For athletic trainers working these events, it can be an extremely rewarding experience or it can be an absolute nightmare. This day was one of the latter. Not only was I becoming accustomed to a new work setting, but we as a staff were working out of a temporary athletic training room. Our facility was undergoing renovations and we had to relocate for the entire year. This also meant that the university had to use 2 practice fields for purposes related to the construction. There was no way that this last camp could take place at our facility. We were expecting well over 300 student athletes. Add in the parents, friends, and coaches that were joining them and we were predicting close to 700 people. In order to accommodate this large number, we had no choice but to move the camp to an off-site location. We were familiar with the site but it was not ideal for a football camp of this size. We made it through the morning session with no real issues. Then the afternoon session began.

My job during the afternoon session was to make sure that all of our hydration stations were fully stocked as the temperature was increasing rapidly. We experienced thunderstorms the night before and the humidity was unbearable. As the afternoon dragged on, my golf cart soon became transportation for several athletes that were experiencing heat-related issues. That number quickly elevated and our undersized athletic training room soon looked like a triage unit with athletes occupying every inch of space. A staff athletic trainer and I were frantically cooling down and hydrating everyone there. The numbers were slightly overwhelming at points during that afternoon. Most of them were able to recover after they were taken out of the heat and hydrated, all but one. This student athlete was an offensive lineman who had walked into the athletic training room with his father reporting nausea and light-headedness. As we hydrated him and monitored his vital signs, he began to slowly deteriorate. He began having full body cramps, ceased sweating, and began to become disoriented. We submerged this athlete in an ice bath and continued to monitor him until he slowly started to recover. I spent a good amount of time speaking with him and his father as he went through this recovery process. He was able to improve enough to walk out of the athletic training room that day. Although the circumstances weren't ideal, I felt that I had done my best.

REFLECTION

To be honest, I had forgotten about this incident as I did not think it was that serious of a situation. The thing I remember the most from that day was how awful it was to set-up and operate efficiently at the off-site location. It wasn't until the following June when I was helping with incoming freshman physicals that I was reminded. I was standing in the athletic training room when I was bear-hugged from behind. I turned and expected to see one of my current lineman messing around as they usually would have done. They weren't there. It was the student athlete from the previous summer. He immediately turned to his fellow incoming freshman and said, "This is the guy that saved my life." This took me completely by surprise. I had no idea that we were recruiting him or that he had signed with us to play football. That moment stands above most experiences I have had as a certified athletic trainer. I know that he was far from the point of losing his life that day; however, in the eyes of that

17-year-old kid I was the one helping him at his lowest point. As we spent the next 4 years together I repeatedly explained to him that he was never really in any danger. He doesn't care. He just enjoys telling people about the day I saved his life.

Noncontact Knee Dislocation

Tim Dunlavey, MS, LAT, ATC

Key Terms

Noncontact Knee Dislocation | Immediate Management of a Knee Dislocation

A sophomore offensive lineman was jogging off of the practice field with the rest of his Division I college football team following a noncontact summer conditioning session. This was a simple task he had done a million times before, but when he made one wrong step, this simple task turned into a medical emergency.

True Story #22

While jogging off the practice field following a summer conditioning session, an offensive lineman attempted to jump around a teammate. This was something the very athletic football player had done several times before. Unfortunately, as he landed, the edge of his foot struck perfectly on the edge of the track and grass. This uneven surface caused him to lose his balance and he dislocated his knee posterolaterally (tibia dislocated posterior and lateral in relation to the femur). The certified athletic trainers that were covering the conditioning session attended to him immediately. As we approached the injured athlete we immediately noticed the obvious deformity of his leg. The deformity could have been the result of a distal femur fracture, proximal tibial fracture or a knee dislocation. Regardless of the actual diagnosis we knew right away that he would need to be transported via ambulance to the hospital. One of the certified athletic trainers called 911 to get an ambulance and then began controlling the rest of the team in an effort to keep them calm and away from the scene. Another certified athletic trainer began to evaluate the injured athlete. There was an obvious posterolateral protrusion without any bleeding. After careful palpation it was determined that the knee had dislocated with the tibia, now posterior and lateral in relation to the femur. The certified athletic trainer continued his evaluation assessing the neurovascular integrity of the leg. There was a palpable pedal pulse but it was diminished compared bilaterally. The distal sensation was also noticeable but slightly diminished compared bilaterally. At this point there was no need to assess any range of motion. The medical staff began to split the leg to prepare to transport the student athlete to the hospital. As we began to splint his leg with a vacuum splint while continuing to monitor his distal pulses, our team orthopedic surgeon happened to be in the building next door and rushed over. The surgeon arrived, confirmed our posterolateral dislocation assessment and decided that it was appropriate to attempt a reduction on the field since the neurovascular structures were clearly being compromised. The reduction was successful and the sensations and pulses immediately returned to normal. His ankle range of motion was within normal limits, but again, no reason to assess the range of motion at the knee. The vacuum splint was reapplied and the athlete was then transported via ambulance to the hospital for further examination.

Following ankle-brachial index tests, doppler scans, magnetic resonance imaging, and X-rays the final diagnosis was:

- Grade 3 anterior cruciate ligament
- Grade 3 posterior cruciate ligament
- Grade 3 medial collateral ligament
- Medial meniscal tear
- No fractures
- No neurovascular compromise

The reconstructive surgery was performed a week later with a complete return to play 10 months later.

REFLECTION

The great immediate care for this catastrophic injury was paramount to the great outcome for this athlete. Proper assessment and management of a knee dislocation significantly increases the chances of a favorable outcome. Like in any medical emergency, it is important for the certified athletic trainers to remain calm, manage the appropriate care for the athlete, and also manage anyone else at the scene.

RESPONDING TO AN EMERGENCY SITUATION
QUICK DECISIONS MAKE FOR POSITIVE OUTCOMES

Tim Giel, MS, LAT, ATC

KEY TERMS
Emergency Action Plan | Facial Bone Anatomy | Signs of Shock

This true story is one where, as an athletic trainer, you must be prepared for anything to happen at any time. Whether it is practice, scrimmage or game situation, severe injuries often do occur when you least expect it and at the most inopportune time and place. Your ability as an athletic trainer to be able to react and correctly handle each situation can be the difference in a negative or positive outcome. In this situation, not only was our emergency action plan (EAP) put into use, but our knowledge of anatomy and emergency procedures were critical in this case.

When approaching this athlete, the gross disfigurement was apparent. Being able to move past that and treat this emergency situation was critical in having a positive outcome. Was the eye intact? How do I examine the integrity of the eye? Keeping the athlete from going into shock, checking his neurological status, vital signs, etc. How do I assess the injury without risking further injury? Making sure surrounding athletes and coaches are okay, how to remove the athlete from the field? Should we remove the athlete from the field? Do I contact parents first or get emergency medical services (EMS) rolling?

These were just a few of the decisions that had to be made and made quickly.

TRUE STORY #23

While watching an intersquad boys' soccer scrimmage, one of our forwards received a pass and was dribbling toward the goal. Our goalie came out to make a diving save as our forward was kicking the ball. The forward made contact with the ball and also with our goalies face during his follow-through. The goalie went down grasping his face. As I approached I could see quite a bit of blood and disfigurement.

His nose was pushed off to the right, there was a rather large laceration under his left eye, and I could see that the left zygomatic arch was fractured.

Upon examination, the patient was coherent but in quite a bit of discomfort. Vital signs were good. We were able to stop the bleeding rather easily, which was surprising considering the amount of disfigurement of his nose and the size of the laceration under his eye. Patient had normal jaw movement and all his teeth were intact. His eye had almost immediately swollen shut but the patient still had good vision. He had no neck or spinal pain but we put on a collar just in case.

We attempted to lie the patient down but that proved to be uncomfortable for him and it began to restrict his breathing. The nose was still bleeding, but it was all draining into his sinus cavities and down his throat.

Being that the patient was a minor, we called the family and the patient's mother insisted we do not call for the ambulance until she arrived. With that decision made, we also needed to remove the athlete from the field because the only access to this field was a dirt path and it was better for us to navigate this path with our all-terrain vehicle than to try and get the ambulance and parent to the field. Once the patient's mother saw the disfigurement and the severity of the injury we called the ambulance for transport.

At the hospital, the X-rays showed fractures of the zygomatic arch, orbital socket, lacrimal bone as well as the nasal bone.

During reconstructive surgery they had to rebuild the eye socket, and the zygomatic arch as well as his sinus cavities.

Patient had surgery in August and the surgeon allowed the patient to return to sports in January.

REFLECTION

Our concerns for this patient were many. Immediately, we needed to take care of bleeding from the nose and the laceration. Secondly, because of the location of the injury, we were concerned about maintaining an airway, his vision, and the patient going into shock as well as the severity of the fractures. We did not want to move him too much because we did not know the position of the bones after they were fractured. That also made it difficult to stop the bleeding because we could not apply direct pressure over the laceration. Attempting to lay the patient down made it very uncomfortable for him. It increased the pressure in the sinuses and made it difficult for him to breathe. We found a semireclined position to be the most comfortable for him. The family lived only minutes away from the school and the parents' insistence of seeing the student first only delayed our emergency response by a few minutes.

Practicing our EAP only weeks before also assisted in this situation. Everyone knew their role and what they needed to do to have a successful outcome.

Our relationship with the team physician and EMS crew also proved very beneficial because we were able to alert the physician and EMS to the injury and they knew what to expect upon their arrival. The physician was able to have the appropriate medical staff in the emergency room to meet the patient upon their arrival.

Domain IV

Treatment and Rehabilitation

LEGAL RISK IN RETURN-TO-PLAY FOR A SOFTBALL PITCHER

Timothy J. Henry, PhD, ATC

KEY TERMS

Return-to-Play | Liability | Negligence

A senior collegiate softball player injures the clavicle on her throwing arm while pitching in preseason practice. The young lady is evaluated by the athletic trainer and describes hearing and feeling a "pop in the collarbone" of her throwing arm. She does not report any previous history of injury to the injured limb. The athlete is referred to the team physician who, after clinical examination and imaging, diagnoses her with a right clavicle fracture. The team physician tells the athlete and her parents that she will not be able to participate in throwing activities for a minimum of 4 to 6 weeks. The athlete will receive a follow-up X-ray at 4 weeks postinjury.

TRUE STORY #24

Following the diagnoses and the 4 to 6 week return-to-play timeline, the softball player is very unhappy and frustrated. She does not want to miss any playing time during the season since she is a senior and she does not have the option to redshirt.

During the first 2 weeks following the injury, the athlete is compliant with the physician and athletic trainer and participates in light cardiovascular conditioning as directed by the athletic trainer. Approximately 2 weeks following injury, the athlete approaches the athletic trainer and states that her arm "feels fine and that she is ready to begin throwing again." The athletic trainer attempts to explain to the athlete that, while it is great that your clavicle and arm feel fine, the healing process for a fracture of the clavicle takes a minimum of 4 weeks to get to the point where the bone is stable and strong enough for higher intensity rehabilitation and progression to throwing. Three weeks postinjury, the athlete and her parents demand an appointment with the team physician in order to gain clearance to participate in full softball

Gorse KM, Feld F, Blanc RO, eds.
True Stories From the Athletic Training Room (pp 89-102).
© 2018 SLACK Incorporated.

activities. At the appointment with the physician, the parents and athlete state that she is "fully healed, has no pain in the clavicle area and full range of motion in her throwing arm." The parents feel that there is no reason for her to be restricted from full participation.

The team physician explains, once again, that although everything feels and looks great, the healing process for the clavicle is not yet complete. The physician also explains that by returning to participation, specifically throwing, too soon the athlete is at risk of refracturing the clavicle. The parents and athlete are adamant that she is fine and they are very upset that the physician and athletic trainer are preventing her from returning and causing her to miss her senior season. After the conversation, the team physician agrees to a follow-up X-ray (at the 3-week postinjury mark). The X-ray reveals that the clavicle was not fully healed and that it is not safe for the athlete to return to pitching at the current time. The athletes and parents are extremely frustrated and unhappy that she is not cleared for participation. The team physician agrees to another X-ray at the 4-week mark.

At the 4 week appointment, the athlete and parents again are adamant that she is fine and she is more than ready to begin throwing again. The physician obtains the X-ray and after consultation with a radiologist, agrees that there is sufficient healing of the clavicle to begin more intense rehabilitation and a return to throwing program. The athlete is told that the progression for complete return to throwing will take 2 to 3 weeks and she should be ready for game participation at the 6 to 7 week postinjury mark. Once again, the athlete and her parents feel as though she should be able to fully participate immediately and that she does not need the additional 2 to 3 weeks of progression. The athletic trainer and physician agree that she will need to complete a functional progression under the supervision of the athletic trainer prior to full return-to-play. This is explained to the athlete and parents and, although unhappy, they agree to work with the athletic trainer on the rehabilitation and progression. This meeting occurred on a Friday and the athlete agreed to return the following Monday to begin the rehabilitation.

On the following Monday, the athlete returned to the athletic trainer and stated, "I think I rebroke my collarbone." The athletic trainer asks her the mechanism of injury and she states that she was pitching to one of her friends over the weekend and it popped again. The athletic trainer evaluates the injury and agrees that she may have refractured the clavicle. An X-ray confirms that she did indeed refracture the clavicle. At this point, the physician notifies her that she will need a minimum of 6 to 8 weeks to heal, wiping out the remainder of her senior softball season.

Approximately one month later the athletic trainer and team physician receive notice from the university legal counsel that they have been named in a suit against the University by the athlete. The charges allege that the team physician and athletic trainer were negligent in treating the athlete and allowed her to return to play too soon following her initial clavicle fracture.

The team physician and athletic trainer were extremely surprised at the lawsuit considering the athlete and her parents alleged that she was ready to return at least 2 weeks prior to the point where she received medical clearance to begin her functional rehabilitation and throwing progression. The parents were very unhappy that she didn't receive clearance to return as early as 2 weeks following the initial injury.

After months of discovery, conversations with legal counsel and depositions the insurance company representing the university settled with the family on a modest monetary sum. The insurance company representing the university believed it would be more cost effective to settle with the family and fund the settlement than to go through the entire process of a trial. The settlement included no admission of negligence on the part of the team physician or athletic trainer.

REFLECTION

Upon reflection, a number of important points become apparent. The first point is that although the physician and athletic trainer felt as though they were accommodating the wishes of the athlete and parents by allowing the athlete to return to softball as early as possible, in reality, they potentially compromised their own professional well-being by allowing the earliest possible return. Secondly, this case reminds us of the importance of reinforcing physician orders with athletes. The softball player in this story received orders from the physician on a Friday that she would begin her functional rehabilitation on the following Monday. She was then injured while working out on her own over the weekend. It would have been wise for the athletic trainer to reinforce with the athlete that she is not to begin her own functional activities over the weekend and that she should be working with the athletic trainer on her rehabilitation. Thirdly, this case is an important reminder that athletes and parents can sometimes act irrationally in cases of injury. Even though the family had no issue in advocating for an early return-to-play, they were not hesitant to "throw the medical team under the bus" after the reinjury.

The take home message from this true story is that it is imperative that the health care team always follow established guidelines, policies, and procedures regarding return-to-play decisions and documentation. The health care team cannot bow to pressure exerted from athletes, parents, coaches, etc. to return an athlete to play prior to full tissue healing and the completion of a comprehensive functional progression. In today's world of increased litigation, the athletic trainer and entire health care team must always remain cognizant of following established protocols to minimize legal risk.

WHAT IS YOUR INFLUENCE?

Larry Cooper, MS, LAT, ATC

KEY TERMS

Communication | Documentation | Relationships

When you work with athletes, you want to have the ability to make a difference in their lives. It is often difficult to gauge your level of influences to keep moving forward. Hopefully, at some point, you will get some feedback that will show you had a positive influence, but sometimes you get feedback suggesting you need to try a little harder or change your delivery method.

TRUE STORY #25

I had just changed schools and was starting in August as a teacher and athletic trainer. There were some very enthusiastic students enrolled in my sports medicine course. Many of them were also athletes which gave them opportunities for immediate feedback of information and principles taught in class, sometimes that very same day. In March, after 7 months with this new group of students and athletes, the spring season started. There were 3 or 4 from the sports medicine class that were soccer players and starters. At an away game, one of these young ladies injured her ankle. The opposing athletic trainer called me and alerted me of the injury which then allowed me to call the parents of the injured student. I shared with them that it appeared to be a Grade 1 inversion ankle sprain, something that we deal with on a regular basis and that I will re-examine her in the morning. I gave them home instructions to keep the ankle level or elevated, ice the ankle for no more than 10 minutes, and then let the skin return to normal temperature before reapplying the ice. They could repeat this as many times as they could but there wasn't any need to wake her from her sleep to do so. I felt good knowing that the injured athlete, also a student in the sports medicine class, would have known how to care for the injury and that her parents were instructed and very responsive to my suggestions.

The next morning, as suggested, I was to meet her in the athletic training room before homeroom. She was waiting for me in usual athlete apparel, sweatpants and sweatshirt, but I could see a hint of an ace wrap on the injured ankle, no big deal, but she did have crutches. I asked if she went for X-rays. She hadn't, but she borrowed them from a neighbor. I proceeded to ask her if she had an increase in pain and that was the reason for the use of crutches to which she replied, "No, just some major swelling." As she pulled up her sweatpants, I was absolutely stunned at the size of her ankle. Her ankle had swollen to almost 3 times the normal size. Typically, during my evaluation, there are a series of standard questions I ask all athletes; however, this was not a normal situation. She did not have any vascular or neurological deficits, but there was a loss of range of movement, a deformity, some discoloration, and massive amounts of swelling, although there was not an increase in pain. Obviously, this was not a normal ankle injury situation and I needed to get a full medical history, leaving no rock unturned.

It did not take long until I found the culprit for the massive swelling. The standard questions led me down the path of home care and what she did. It turns out that my influence as a teacher and athletic trainer paled in comparison to her coach. Coach A for reasons of confidentiality, was from South America and they handled injuries slightly different than we did. He had instructed her and her parents to take a brick and put it in the oven at 400° for 30 minutes. Then take that brick out, wrap it into a towel and then wrap that towel around the injured ankle all evening. When she woke up, her ankle had swollen to 3 times the original size, and she stated that the swelling had actually gone down since she removed the towel that contained the brick. Unfortunately, this young lady's season ended with that injury, not because of the actual injury but because of the swelling. It took over 6 weeks for her ankle to return to the point that she could perform any running or soccer skills.

REFLECTION

This situation made me increase my efforts to connect with student athletes and educate the coaches on how to properly handle injuries if I wasn't present. It also made me increase my efforts to educate the parents on the skill set of the athletic trainer and also proper injury management while their sons and daughters are at home. While it increased my workload, as well as time and effort on the job, it was well worth the effort to avoid a similar situation in the future.

BALLISTIC TRAUMA IN A COLLEGIATE FOOTBALL STUDENT ATHLETE

Giampietro L. Vairo, PhD, LAT, ATC

KEY TERMS

Ballistic Trauma | Gunshot Wound | Upper Extremity

Athletic trainers routinely clinically evaluate, diagnose, treat, and rehabilitate neuromusculoskeletal injuries related to participation in sports and athletic activities; however, occasionally, athletic trainers are also called upon to apply these same practice domain skills to clinical conditions that stem from other, sometimes unusual, mechanisms of injury. This true story reflects an unusual experience while working as a young professional in a National Collegiate Athletic Association Division I intercollegiate athletics setting. It also briefly describes some of the applicable treatment and rehabilitation techniques employed to manage this unique patient case while also stressing the need for athletic trainers to be culturally competent caregivers when interacting with any and all patients. The integration of an evolving knowledge base, mastered psychomotor skills, and a compassionate approach sets the groundwork for an athletic trainer that is well poised to successfully handle the wide-ranging types of scenarios that he or she may face in what is often a challenging career in the allied health sciences.

TRUE STORY #26

In the second year of my first full-time job an assistant athletic trainer with a National Collegiate Athletic Association Division I football program, I had been exposed to myriad of different clinical conditions, treated a spectrum of student athletes, and worked alongside a multitude of trailblazers in the field of sports medicine. In this capacity, and in consultation with the head athletic trainer, and supervising team physician, I was tasked with coordinating the rehabilitative plans of care for our football student athletes. While in this position, I had experienced a number of rare and unusual cases that spanned from a pilonidal abscess to a fractured scapula. Nothing prepared me for the most unpredictable and exceptional event I would ever treat as an athletic trainer, which was ballistic trauma, or a gunshot wound.

I recall getting to work one early morning and the head athletic trainer informing me that the in the late night hours of the preceding evening, a football student athlete fell victim to a shooting. The student athlete, who was a highly recruited scholarship player, suffered a gunshot wound to the shoulder and was scheduled to undergo subsequent trauma surgery. It was explained to me that the student athlete would be released from the hospital following initial trauma management and that we, as an athletic training and sports medicine staff, would be providing his follow-up care as appropriate unless otherwise noted since specifics of the event were still developing.

Without firsthand knowledge of the injury, it was described as substantial given that it occurred at close proximity to the firearm, and the entrance wound was adjacent to the branches of the brachial plexus. Furthermore, it was communicated that damage to delicate adjacent neurovascular structures and soft tissue was extensive and that the exit wound coursed through the distal third of the arm. With no concrete foundation for the pathoetiology and sequelae of ballistic trauma, all this information was challenging to process. Further complications from an operations standpoint involved claims that the incident revolved around alleged illegal activity.

While my athletic training education and early professional experiences provided me with the fundamental basis to deliver a sound prescribed rehabilitative paradigm to restore functional capacity of the injured upper extremity, I was unaware of how and why the trauma surgeon employed the operative techniques he did which contributed to the specific type of wound and related management strategies we would apply in our practice setting. This peaked my interest and curiosity for my own knowledge as well as the clinical education of athletic training students that I was supervising in fieldwork. Through discussions with our supervising team physician and a survey of the literature, I came to discover classification systems and related management of ballistic trauma. This knowledge was primarily focused on the patterns for tissue injury associated with high, intermediate, and low velocity round gunshot wounds.

High velocity rounds are mostly associated with military grade assault or hunting rifles and result in wounds that measure greater than 10 cm which cause them to be highly susceptible to infection. High velocity rounds also have the propensity to drag debris (typically clothing) through the intermediary tissues anchored by the entrance and exit wounds, which may require wide excision and possibly fasciotomy necessary for debridement of foreign material, and necrotic tissue.

Intermediate velocity rounds usually originate from shotguns and yield variable wound sizes often dependent upon distance from the target and the size of the bullet. Low velocity rounds, as was the situation with this patient case, commonly result in wound sizes that range from approximately 1 to 10 cm. This low velocity type of round is less likely to require surgical debridement unless the shot occurs at close range, which is what this patient experienced and added to the complexity of his case. Based on his wound, routine cleansing and dressing of the area with sterile materials was necessary due to the potential vulnerability for tetanus, anaerobic bacterial infection, and gas gangrene; therefore, our cutaneous and subcutaneous wound care approach for managing this case in an athletic training facility was adapted to closely parallel the standards of a wound clinic.

Given the unique peripheral circumstances associated with this case, the extent of care provided was relatively short-term since the student athlete and institution parted ways; nonetheless, the student athlete made a successful medical recovery, regained functional capacity of his arm, and went on to finish his collegiate playing career at another university. Furthermore, he also enjoyed a period as a professional athlete.

REFLECTION

This distinctive experience was certainly one that most athletic trainers may not encounter in their professional practice; however, it definitely provided me with an opportunity to broaden my clinical knowledge base, specifically as it applied to the examination and treatment of neuromusculoskeletal injuries. This is especially applicable to contemporary athletic training education and practice given the emerging prevalence of athletic trainers in the military and other related government service agencies like law enforcement, which may yield exposures to these types of nontraditional scenarios. Moreover, this clinical case provided me with an opportunity to further develop and sharpen my cultural competence skills, which helped bolster my capability to work with diverse patient populations.

Consequently, this afforded me the occasion to learn different values, attitudes, behaviors, and styles of communication that affect and shape an individual's choices and responses. Specifically, it contributed to my personal growth as an individual, and clinician, which in the years following, provided a platform for creating a culturally sensitive environment that improved the services I provided to the diverse patient population I worked with. In hindsight, this very uncommon. This brief situation has had a long-lasting impact on me in a multitude of ways. Primarily, it has made me ever more grateful for the many and wide-ranging opportunities that the profession of athletic training has delivered, thereby contributing to my development as a clinician, scientist, and citizen of society.

NECK INJURY WITH AN UNEXPECTED OUTCOME

Gaetano Sanchioli MS, LAT, ATC, PES

KEY TERMS

Scoliosis | Neuropraxia | Astrocytoma

An athlete presented with neck and back pain a week after a tackling event during a middle school football practice. After going to the emergency room, he had not been to practice since the incident. The coach asked that he seek treatment prior to returning to the field.

After the initial evaluation, it was noted that he had severe scoliosis, however, he also had point tenderness in his lower cervical and upper thoracic spine. The athlete was under the care of a physician who was monitoring the scoliosis currently.

TRUE STORY #27

A middle school athlete came to the athletic training room due to neck and back pain that was caused by a collision the prior week during a football game. He was seen in the emergency room and told to rest. On the advice of his coach, the athlete came to the training room seeking help to reduce the pain and strengthen the area so he could return to football.

During the initial evaluation, it was noted that he had issues with scoliosis in the past and was under the care of a physician who was monitoring its progression. His neck displayed full range of motion with no areas of point tenderness in the upper cervical. Strength was 4/5 in all directions and neck movement caused minimal discomfort. It was noted, however, that he was point tender along the midline from C6 through T3. He also complained of generalized shoulder and upper back pain, primarily on the right side both with and without movement. I did not want to progress with any therapy at this point until advised by his physician. He had an upcoming appointment so the plan was to talk to the physician and request permission to start exercise.

The visit with the physician raised some concerns with the football injury because his pain wasn't going away and his scoliosis had increased from 11 to 44 degrees in the 3 months prior to this visit. He was scheduled for a follow-up with another specialist in the coming weeks, but was allowed to begin stretching and light strengthening within the limits of comfort. At that time, we began posture exercise on the physioball with pelvic stabilization and tilting, arm and leg movements, and core strengthening.

When he returned to the specialist, he underwent further testing including a computerized tomography scan and magnetic resonance imaging. It was found that he had a tumor growing from the spinal cord and all exercise was discontinued until a biopsy could be completed.

The biopsy results determined that this athlete had an astrocytoma and more testing was required to determine if it was benign or malignant. It was determined that the tumor was Stage I and the plan was to remove as much of the tumor as possible at that time.

Due to the trauma of the surgery, he was left with monoplegia of the lower right extremity and sensory deficit of the left lower extremity. It was expected that normal function would return in time and he was given time to recover from the surgery and begin physical therapy.

After several weeks of physical therapy, the father asked if I could work with his son in addition to the regular therapy sessions. After receiving a physician's script, we began passive, active, and active assistive range of motion of his hip, knee, ankle and toes. The paralysis and atrophy had caused contractures and weakness that made movement painful. Russian stimulation was utilized for muscle re-education along with proprioceptive neuromuscular facilitation stretching and massage.

As he improved, we progressed to active assistive and manual progressive resistive exercises for all the joints of the lower extremity. We also continued with the physioball and core exercises which incorporated the core and lower extremity.

After several months of therapy, 3 to 4 days a week, he was discontinued from the cane as his walking was improving, though he still had a mild drop foot. Normal sensation returned to the extremity and strength continued to improve. He was eager to play baseball with his friends in the spring and that was his main goal at that time.

As his improvement continued, we progressed to lifting weights and doing most of the workouts on the physioball. In addition to swimming, kickboard, and aerobics, we also incorporated games in the pool such as basketball and shallow and deep water running. He began jogging and running on dry land, which at times caused discomfort, so the pool was a helpful change.

In April, he was cleared to participate in sports as tolerated. His only disability was full sprinting with a limp. His ankle was supported with ankle taping for the drop foot and functional knee brace. At times, he would have anterior knee pain with increased activity level so he was given extra rest when needed while continuing to rehabilitate strength and flexibility. He was also given extra rest days as he would fatigue more quickly.

Two years after the initial evaluation, this athlete underwent radiation on the tumor. He continued to play baseball through high school and did rehab 2 to 3 times per week depending on time. He has continued to have periodic scans and testing to check on the progression of the tumor which has been minimal.

REFLECTION

In looking back on this case, I would say that the most important thing to take from this is to never assume things are what they appear to be. A thorough history and physical evaluation in every case is important and always be prepared to refer when the results aren't adding up.

Communication with the physician is important to assure proper care. In this case, pushing the therapy too much may have had detrimental results. His physicians were very much in favor of being as active as possible as long as it was tolerable.

Athletes are not immune to these types of disabilities, but know your boundaries. Communication with the physical therapy was helpful so we were not duplicating treatments and the athlete was able to get the most out of both athletic trainer and physical therapy sessions. The physical therapist and I were able to work together and learn from each other and it became a great team effort.

TIGER PRIDE AND PERSEVERANCE

Randy McGuire, MS, ATC, LAT

KEY TERMS

Closed Fracture | Antibiotic Rod | Prosthesis

During a home National Association of Intercollegiate Athletics (NAIA) college football game on October 18, 2014, a starting defensive back was engaged with the opponent's gunner on a punt return when he was collided into resulting in a closed fracture to the right tibia and fibula. The athletic training staff and orthopedic surgeon immediately ran onto the field to begin evaluation and treatment. Deformity was obvious and some diminished neurologic response was noted. Emergency medical services was summoned onto the field and the right leg was placed in a splint. The athlete was then transported to a local hospital for further examination and radiological testing. That evening, the orthopedic surgeon performed intramedullary nail fixation of the tibia. It was determined that the fibula would heal over time and no surgical intervention was required.

TRUE STORY #28

The athlete returned to campus following a short recovery at home and began treatment and rehabilitation in the athletic training room. He had diminished sensation on the lateral aspect of the lower leg and foot along with very minimal range of motion in the ankle and toes with significant effusion. A plan was initiated, working on range of motion of the entire limb from hip to toes. The plan also focused on hip and knee strengthening exercises. He continued on this program until semesters' end and continued at home during the holiday break. Upon his return to school for the spring semester, the plan was adjusted and new goals set. He also began rehabilitation at a local physical therapy clinic in conjunction with his athletic training room rehabilitation. In physical therapy sessions, they implemented joint mobilizations of the foot and ankle and pool workouts.

During a routine follow-up appointment with the surgeon it was determined there was a lack of bone union and a bone stimulator was provided for the athlete. He continued struggling with sensation and movement in the ankle and foot. The athlete decided to finish the semester at home and continue rehabilitation due to convenience and mobility issues.

Following another physician follow-up appointment, a second surgery was set for May 5, 2015 due to the nonunion right ankle manipulation, tibial exchange of the rod, and bone graft with demineralized bone matrix (DePuy Synthes) was performed. Postsurgery rehabilitation was continued at a physical therapy clinic in his hometown.

He began experiencing pain and swelling during these sessions in late May and June. The athlete went to a surgeon at home and it was determined a staph infection had developed and a third surgery in early July was conducted in which the leg was cleaned and the tibial rod was removed and replaced with an antibiotic rod. Rehabilitation was halted postsurgery and the athlete was placed on oral antibiotics and crutches. Later that summer, a fourth surgery was indicated to remove the antibiotic rod and replace it with a titanium rod. Rehabilitation began postsurgery with progression toward weight bearing activities.

Unfortunately, the infection returned and subsequently 4 more surgeries were performed over the next 3 months to remove tissue decay and infection. Vacuum wound treatment was used in each of these procedures. In November the athlete was given the choice to continue treatments or consider amputation just below the right knee. After much thought and prayer it was decided that surgery number 9 would be amputation on November 16, 2015, about and a year and a month from the date of injury.

The athlete returned to campus for the spring semester of 2016 with a newly fitted prosthesis and began winter weights with a goal of returning to play. The prosthetic had a solid ankle cushioned heal (SACH) foot which permitted functional activity levels. He began physical therapy in addition to the weights in March with the primary focus on core, quad eccentrics, agility and closed-chain activities. He participated in spring football practice in limited contact drills. The athlete experienced some difficulty in opening the hips and turning as if covering a receiver because the prosthesis was turning at the insertion point of the leg. Adjustment of the leg and prosthetic continued throughout the remaining of spring practice. In late April, the athlete was fitted with a prosthesis with a sports performance blade to use solely for activities and used this during the summer in preparation for the fall season. Summer activity included an emphasis on hip rehabilitation, core strength, and agilities along with team summer workouts.

Returning to full participation in the fall of 2016 did provide some challenge, aside from the many that were overcome to this point. The athlete began to suffer some skin irritation and breakdown which led to burning and phantom pain at the amputation site. We noticed this occurred on particularly hot days on the turf so we limited reps and sprayed with cold water to alleviate this pain. He was referred back to get the prosthetic socket refitted which proved very beneficial but he missed one varsity game due to this repair. To help with traction of the blade, the bottom of a spiked shoe was removed and taped to the blade to provide traction. I personally never envisioned taping a prosthetic blade as part of my skills set. The athlete experienced a stress reaction to the pubic bone toward the end of the season but we are not sure of its relationship to overcompensation or increased hip rehabilitation over the year. The NAIA follows National Collegiate Athletic Association rules so I contacted an NCAA official who oversees replays, because he is a personal friend, to find out if there were any rules and regulations on prosthetic devices being used, particularly the blade. He contacted one of the National Collegiate Athletic Association Football Rules Committee members and it was determined all we had to do was cover the edges with tape and pad the exposed metal piece. I then contacted our conference commissioner to instruct the NAIA officials on their ruling. Lastly, the athlete participated in 4 junior varsity games as a cornerback and even had an interception in his first game back in action. He dressed in all of the varsity games except the one in which the prosthetic was being repaired and recorded 1 solo tackle and returned 4 kickoffs for a 24.5 yard average the largest being 41 yards.

REFLECTION

The student athlete was able to overcome a traumatic negative experience and turn it into a positive. His ability to set goals and incorporate an unparalleled work ethic to reach them is something to be greatly admired. The experience he went through had a great impact on those around him, especially his teammates. They were able to see firsthand what hard work and dedication can accomplish. A number of his teammates expressed to me how, when things got tough physically or mentally in conditioning, practice, or games, his influence pushed them to succeed. In football, and sports in general, there are many slogans used for motivation to strive for success and sometimes they fall on deaf ears. This experience provided a chance to witness pride and perseverance on a daily basis.

Domain V

Organizational and Professional
Health and Well-being

CATASTROPHIC EVENTS AFFECT ALL INVOLVED

Paul A. Cacolice, PhD, LAT, ATC, CSCS

KEY TERMS

Mental Health | Catastrophic Injury | Care Provider as a Patient

During my first season as the sole athletic trainer for a team, I had done my best to document and practice an effective and efficient emergency action plan (EAP) during the offseason. The coaching staff, rink personnel, gameday staff, and town emergency medical services representatives had practiced procedures for care and extrication of injured athletes during preseason, and we verbally reviewed the steps and hand signals before each game with all parties and visiting team representatives. As we had utilized town services for transportation for limb injuries several times during the season, we thought we had prepared for anything, like a well-oiled machine.

TRUE STORY #29

The night started out as a challenge and became progressively worse. After 2 periods of a junior hockey game, I had evaluated an athlete for a likely tibia-fibula fracture with transportation to the nearest hospital emergency room. Another athlete was immobilized and transported by his parents to the emergency room for a grossly sprained acromioclavicular joint. To compound the professional stress, the visiting team athletic trainer was unable to accompany their team to this game and I was asked to provide care for both teams. The rink also seemed extra cold with the air near ice level at 19°F. As the sole athletic trainer covering a very busy event, I was looking forward to the end of the game, returning home and warming myself up.

At the start of the third period, the home team was on the power play with a fresh and very slick sheet of ice. A slap shot from the point caught the defending athlete at the base of his helmet as he turned his head. The defender let out an interjection,

Gorse KM, Feld F, Blanc RO, eds.
True Stories From the Athletic Training Room (pp 105-127).
© 2018 SLACK Incorporated.

stopped midway through a second interjection and fell to the ice face down. The play was immediately stopped by players on both teams and the players quickly escorted me onto the ice.

As I slid towards athlete, I could hear his loud breathing while lying unconscious and face down on the ice. Within seconds, I signaled the town police officer stationed at the rink to assist in anticipation of a log roll technique. While I was assessing the athlete, the officer contacted the town emergency medical services, requesting timely arrival of paramedics. Immediate assessment of the athlete and his labored breathing suggested that his condition could deteriorate rapidly. As such, we signaled for rink personnel to fulfill their roles. The Zamboni (Frank J. Zamboni & Co.) was moved from the tunnel to allow for direct access to the ice surface from the access road for the ambulance. The announcer asked the fans to make their way to the concourse and players to their respective locker rooms. The home coaches and gameday personnel took their places to assist as needed. All previously rehearsed actions were proceeding smoothly, which was fortuitous. Paramedics arrived as the athlete's condition worsened. As a team, we effectively worked to have the athlete immediately removed from the rink and to the local Level 1 trauma center within minutes of incident.

As we managed the scene afterwards, the coaches, rink personnel and I all remarked that we were exhausted, drenched with sweat (in such a cold rink) and assumed we had been working for 20 minutes or so. The scoreboard operator commented that the whole event had taken less than 10 minutes. At this point, the coaches rightly agreed with the referees to postpone the game to a later date.

While this story may be similar to many, the readers may or may not have experienced. What occurred next greatly affected how I practiced for the next 20 plus years.

As tired as we all were, the head coach caught us and brought everyone into the team offices and locker room. Having experienced catastrophic events before, he was aware of what we hadn't planned in our EAP: the postevent response. He had contacted our team counselor (a doctoral student in psychology) who arrived as we reflected on all that occurred. The counselor then met with the team while the head coach brought us all to the team meeting room. As we ordered food, we began to talk as part of the process.

It was very early in the morning when we heard from the emergency room that the athlete was in the Intensive Care Unit, but alive. The team had headed home long ago in groups to watch out for each other. The remaining staff went out to breakfast with the team counselor and assured him that we were as emotionally healthy as possible.

REFLECTION

So often, great detail is generated into an EAP for justified reasons. What is often overlooked; however, is the plan for the care providers during and after a traumatic event. Understanding the stress involved while caring for the injured can often be emotionally traumatic. As such, it should be incorporated into creation of any EAP.

CONFLICT IN THE WORKPLACE

Adam Annaccone, EdD, ATC, CES, PES

KEY TERMS
Conflict | Conflict Management | Collaboration

The workplace is supposed to be a place of collaboration, teamwork, and dedication. This is a place where individuals can bring their own unique talents and interests for the betterment of the organization. In health care, patients and clients rely on this collaboration to ensure the best and most up-to-date medical practices are being utilized to ensure quality treatment and favorable outcomes. The athletic training facility and program is no different and should be held to these high standards.

Unfortunately, when collaboration breaks down, an athletic training facility and program can find itself in a whirlwind of conflict, which can have potentially harmful effects on the patients under our care.

TRUE STORY #30

We all have encountered supervisors or managers whose decisions and policies we may have disagreed with. Often, as athletic trainers, we feel we can perform their job better than they can. For managers, a lack of support may provoke communication breakdown. But imagine you had a supervisor whose decisions went above and beyond just disagreeing with policy and procedure? What if you had a supervisor who none of your coworkers respected and felt was responsible for the downward spiral of the department consisting of conflict and bad decisions? In health care, this creates a poor environment for quality care.

The start of the fall athletic season was fast approaching and as athletic trainers, we were busy taking inventory of supplies, reviewing medical forms, and completing the many checklists we use to ensure everything is in order for when the first athlete steps on campus at a small National Collegiate Athletic Association Division II university. Staff sports medicine meetings were now becoming more frequent (once or twice a week) to foster communication among coworkers and to discuss any potential problems we may encounter before the season begins at the end of summer.

Conflict in our department wasn't uncommon. With so many moving parts and different opinions, some of the best solutions came from conflict or disputes. This particular year started differently though. We noticed in our meetings that as we discuss policy, procedures, and new initiatives, we would leave the meetings hopeful and full of optimism. Unfortunately, we were quickly disappointed as promises and agreements slowly went by the wayside. Eager to start the fall season, many of my coworkers and I were willing to allow some leeway and focus on our specific sport assignments. It was a decision many of us would regret.

As the season started, so did the chaos. We noticed 3 different medical forms were being used for physicals, team physicians were unaware of physical start times, certain athletes could reschedule a missed physical at the health center (which was not permissible according to our policy and procedures) while others were not, and it seemed like all communication between the head athletic trainer and the assistants had stopped. In my 7 years practicing as an athletic trainer, this was by far the most unorganized start to any sports season. My co-workers and I immediately went into crisis management mode to "survive" physicals and get athletes cleared to start pre-season camp. At this point, our team physicians were furious, the health center was overloaded, and coaches were storming around wondering why athletes had not been cleared. Doing what athletic trainers do best, we patched up the wounds the best we could to limit the damage.

Following the disaster of preseason, we had time to reflect and come together as a staff to determine what areas could be improved upon. In our very first meeting, we were shocked to hear our head athletic trainer discuss how happy he or she was with how the preseason process went and he or she felt it was the smoothest preseason yet. We were floored by the complete disregard for the mess we just experienced. My colleagues and I presented areas we felt did not go smoothly and suggestions to improve. Our ideas were met with disingenuous nods of agreement from the head athletic trainer followed by, "I don't think we need to be drastic as everything went just as it should have gone." At the conclusion of the meeting, we were left with more questions than answers. The assistants gathered as a group and decided it was necessary to speak with the head athletic trainer individually to express our concerns and to see if it would foster better communication and recognition for what we felt was a completely unprofessional fall preseason.

Individual meeting after individual meeting, each assistant (again) felt like his or her concerns were not being heard. So it was time for a more aggressive plan. At out next meeting, we would all again express our concerns and bring in the concerns of the team physicians, health center, and coaches. This strategy was again met with complete denial. We found ourselves at a stalemate and (little did we know) things would only get worse.

Week after week we were met with inactivity, disregard for the current state of the program, and suggestion for improvement unheard. Instead of running an effective and efficient health care facility, individualism started to take over as athletic trainers needed to make decisions regarding their specific athletes and sport assignments. Even our team physicians were beginning to question their partnership with the program as it continued to break down. The downward trend continued for the entire year. Instead of working as a team to ensure quality health care, we were doing what we thought was best to "get by." Luckily, the health and safety of our patients were never directly put into question. In retrospect, we were lucky.

REFLECTION

As I reflect on this not-so-impressive year, many thoughts and ideas run through my head. We had a supervisor who, for one reason or another, viewed the operation of the program in a different way than the assistants and team physicians. We would find out later that our head athletic trainer felt threatened by the assistants as if we were all "ganging up" against him or her. Perhaps at the time, if this was communicated to the group, we could have had a serious discussion to help break the wall of division. It was never our intent to make our supervisor feel threatened. In addition, I think our biggest mistake was not expressing our opinions and viewpoints prior to the start of preseason. As I mentioned, we were all eager for sports to start and we allowed that excitement to overshadow potential problems and concerns each of us was experiencing. We allowed our emotions to take control.

Conflict is going to occur in our profession as there are so many variables to running an efficient and effective sports medicine program. While some conflict is beneficial and fosters new ideas and growth, negative conflict (which often is neglected or suppressed) can often bring an entire department to a halt.

DEATH OF AN ATHLETE

Richard Burr, MS, LAT, ATC, CSCS

I had been a head university athletic trainer for about 8 years and thought I had experienced it all. This situation, however, changed how I performed the administration part of my job and the importance of having a multidisciplinary team when dealing with situations. It was a typical winter day, and I had returned home after a long day of practice coverage. Nothing major had happen that day, but little did I know what laid ahead. I was just about to go to bed when the phone rang. The assistant swim coach had called. He informed me that one of the sophomore male swimmers had collapse that evening while playing basketball. Campus police was summoned and performed cardiopulmonary resuscitation but were unable to revive him.

TRUE STORY #31

I was deeply shaken by the news. I knew the athlete briefly, and while I had not treated any of his injuries, he was still a member of "our family". I asked the coach if the athlete was at practice that afternoon. The coach told me he was but was sent back to the dorms by the head coach because he was not feeling good. At the moment, it was difficult to take everything in, but I knew there were many more phone calls to come. I thanked the coach and called the athletic director. He already knew and was dealing with campus police and university administration as well as the head coach.

The athletic director asked me if I was aware of any medical problems with the athlete. The athlete's name did not trigger any memory I had of athletes we had identified as at risk, but knew I would need to review his records. I had never dealt with a death of an athlete before.

We started going thru the list of who had been contacted and saw the parents were en route. We talked about disclosing the news to the team members and how the team would handle death. I informed the athletic director that I would head into the office and meet with the department of student life to see what needed to be done. I would also review the athlete's medical file for any medical conditions. The next call was to the head coach to see how he was doing. He was very upset. I told him I was heading back to the university and if he needed anything to call me there. He was going to the hospital to talk with the parents.

It was a long drive to the office at midnight. I had plenty of time to try and absorb everything going on. Trying to remember college classes on the stages of grief, I realized I would be the person people would come to for help and answers. I needed to try and gather as much information possible to start the process of supporting the "survivors." I met with campus life. They had already contacted residential life and started grief counseling. There would be more counseling sessions set up for the following day. I felt that they were handling things well and I should to let them do their work. The next thing was to review the athlete's records.

I had always been strict about creating medical records on all the athletes during a time when all we had were paper copies of everything. After reviewing preparticipation physicals and medical history, it was clear that the athlete was a normal healthy athlete. I was confused, but realized that sometime we do not know all the answers. I call the athletic director and informed him of my findings. I did inform him that the athlete had left practice early because he was not feeling well. The athletic director asked me what the policy was if an athlete left practice because he was sick. It was our policy that if that happened the head coach was to notify the athletic training room.

The next day was crazy. People were asking questions, university officials contacted me about medical records, and tried to maintain a calm appearance. Student life was counseling the swim team. When the athletic director and I met with the head coach, I informed the head coach of my findings and asked about the previous practice. The head coach felt he was doing the right thing about sending the athlete back to the dorm and did not want to "bother" the athletic training staff. We had a lengthy discussion of emergency action plans and how plans were in place for all sorts of situations, not just extreme emergencies. I stressed that we needed to make sure that we knew everything about the situation as we moved forward. At this point, the coach had informed us that the parents knew that this would happen to their son. In shock, we ask what he was talking about. After long talks with the parents, he informed us that the athlete had a heart condition that the athlete and the family did not want anyone to know, including the family physician. The parents stressed that they wanted their son to get the most out of his life and did not want him to miss out on anything because of his condition. This information was rather difficult to process. Coach had informed us that this information was being presented to university officials as we speak. Even though my emotions were all over the place, I had to maintain a calm exterior for everyone else.

REFLECTION

Looking back on the situation, there were so many things I learned. First, was the realization that it was important to emphasize emergency action plans with coaches and that "emergencies" come in all shapes and sizes. We will never know if the athlete's death could have been prevented. Next, was the importance of paperwork and really sitting down with each new athlete. Medical records are not all encompassing and the reality is that people hide the truth. I also realized that I cannot do everything and to stress the multidisciplinary approach. I also saw how effective and important counseling is. Finally, I realized later how much I also needed counseling afterward to help me deal with everything.

THE VALUE OF BEING PREPARED FOR EMERGENCIES

Keith M. Gorse, EdD, LAT, ATC

KEY TERMS

Emergency Action Plan | Emergency Team Personnel | Transport to Health Care Facility

---

Professional, college, and high school sports teams and organizations dictate policies and practice procedures in case of medical emergencies. Most college sports events require proper emergency personnel to be on the scene in case there is a need for transport to a local emergency health care facility.

TRUE STORY #32

Be prepared! During an emergency, those 2 simple words could possibly mean the difference between proper medical care and negligence.

Professional, college, and high school sports teams and organizations dictate policies and practice procedures in case of medical emergencies. Most college sports events require proper emergency personnel to be on the scene in case there is a need for transport to a local emergency health care facility.

During my first year as the head athletic trainer at Carnegie Mellon University (CMU), a small Division III school in Pittsburgh, I had a short amount of time to update a proper emergency action plan (EAP) for the football facility and game day operations. Everything was going well with the revision of the EAP until I found out that there would not be any emergency medical services (EMS) available for on-site coverage of the CMU home football games. All transport of injured athletes, for both teams, would be handled by campus police using their security van. This van had no secure function for proper transport with stretchers or spine boards.

After finding out about this situation from my athletic director at CMU, I began to question the existing policy that was in place and requested that we change that policy immediately. The 2 reasons I was given for having campus police transport injured athletes was cost and convenience. This practice had been in place for over 15 years for all CMU home football games. We needed to revise the emergency transport policy to make it properly aligned for the type of EAP that was being updated for the football facility and its gameday operations. The CMU athletic department did not want to change this policy at first, but after meeting with the football coaching staff, team physician, and athletic director, we all decided that it would be in the best interest to the program and the athletes to provide proper coverage and transportation in case of a medical emergency. This meeting took place less than 2 weeks prior to the beginning of football preseason camp.

The major road block for having EMS present at all home football games was cost. There was not a lot of money left in the football operating budget at that time and we were not allowed to go over budget. I was required to gather 4 to 5 bids from local ambulance companies in the area, including the city of Pittsburgh EMS. It took nearly the entire 2 weeks before preseason to get all bids in for review. In the end, only one private EMS company came in under budget for their services. With the okay from the athletic administration, I was allowed to set up a contract with that EMS company for the entire football season, which included one preseason scrimmage and 5 football games.

The home preseason scrimmage that took place after the first full week of football camp had our first contracted ever EMS company and ambulance in place for coverage and emergency transport. CMU was scrimmaging with Geneva College and the scrimmage was set up with 2 plays going on at the same time from each of the 40 yard lines towards the end zones. Each team had its first offense going against the other team's second defense.

During the third play, on the side where the Geneva College's first team offense was playing, a Geneva offensive lineman was chop-blocked low below the left knee and his low leg buckled under the force. Because the athletic trainer from Geneva was unable to attend the scrimmage because of home events, I was the only certified athletic trainer on hand to take care of all medical issues.

I ran to the scene of the injury and observed that the Geneva lineman had a compound fracture of both the tibia and fibula of the left leg. Both bones had broken through the skin and his low leg was angled at about 45 degrees. I immediately activated our newly revised EAP and motioned for team physician and EMS to the field for emergency medical assistance. It took less than 12 minutes to properly evaluate, stabilize, splint and get the athlete on a stretcher and into the ambulance which had moved onto the field and was next to the injured player. Once we properly placed the injured athlete into the ambulance, it was a quick transport to the local emergency trauma facility that would be able to handle this injury. Communication to the emergency facility took place before arrival and the athlete was able to bypass normal hospital emergency room protocol and was allowed to go straight to the operating room.

From the time that the injury initially occurred to the time of arriving to the operating room for treatment, less than 30 minutes had elapsed. The Geneva football player had successful surgery to repair both bones and the soft tissue around the area of the injury. He was told by the attending orthopedic surgeon that he would have full recovery and would be able to play football again in the future if he desired to do so.

REFLECTION

Without the revision of the EAP and hiring the EMS company, it is difficult to say how this situation may have turned out. Emergency action plans are important for the full safety of athletes. This includes field safety, proper communication, and emergency transportation availability. The EAP should all be in writing and approved by the medical staff and the athletic administration. Many people think that we have it all in our heads for what we should do in case of a medical emergency, but it all has to be in writing and then properly practiced if it is going to work in the correct manner. Development and revisions of proper EAP for all athletic teams, at any level, should not take a long time to properly put together and get approved. It only takes a few moments of our life to make sports safe. The key thing is to get everyone on the same page and make it work for the benefit of our athletes.

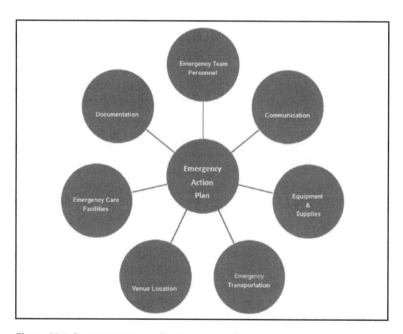

Figure 32-1. Emergency action plan component chart.

AN ATHLETIC TRAINER ON A SCHOOL BOARD

Bill Couts, LAT, ATC

I was a member of a local school board at the same school I had been contracted to work for over 20 years.

TRUE STORY #33

Public service is not much different than our roles as athletic trainers. My foray into politics started when I decided I wanted to work the polls on election days. Not a difficult task to get started, I called some friends and requested write-in votes for inspector of elections. I did that for 2 and a half years. I resigned that position and again called friends for write-in votes when I saw that no one was running for an open seat on my local school board. I was the only successful write-in candidate in the primary elections, leaving me running unopposed in the November general election. During the time between the primaries and the general election, the school district did it is due diligence to determine whether I was eligible to serve as a board member since I was a contracted employee. The state ethics commission found that I was allowed to serve as there was a precedent set in another school district where a contracted school bus driver ran and won a seat on his local school board, but I would have to refrain from any board actions regarding coaches or the athletic director as I had a working relationship with those people. I also had to informed my employer and was required to fill out their conflict of interest and ethics report.

I was sworn in in December and began my 4-year term. I was welcomed by all the current members and we engaged in the normal training provided. Meetings were fairly routine, approving policy changes, education items like field trips, personnel changes, and financials. I abstained from voting or discussing coaches during these sessions. I could discuss how many positions we were going to fill, but not who would fill them.

I am fortunate enough at my school to have multiple certified athletic trainers. We have always planned our schedules around personal activities and my coworkers were very flexible with my scheduled meetings. During my 4-year term, I missed only one meeting. It was a special meeting to hire a new superintendent. District policy allows for phone-in votes in special circumstances. I called in a "yes" vote from the sidelines of a football game.

We had some significant events during my term. These aren't necessarily in chronological order. Negotiations had begun with the teacher's union and they weren't going well. This was just a year or 2 after the "great recession" and money from state and federal sources was dwindling. I was part of the board negotiating team. After many failed attempts at negotiation, we resorted to fact-finding. This is when an arbitrator looks at both sides and sets the ground work for what could be a solution. The fact finding was very much in the districts favor. The union ultimately went on strike after a hard day of work on Labor Day. During the strike, we continued to negotiate and ultimately settled on binding arbitration. I continued to work during this time. Practices and games were scheduled around the picket line so as to minimize the impact on the students. Very few of our coaches were teachers so things were relatively unaffected in the athletic arena. This was probably the most difficult time I had on the board. I won't say that my personal relationships with the district staff were bad, we simply didn't talk about it and kept our professional distance from each other. There were a few teachers who, while passing through hallways, would avoid saying hello, while it stressful, it wasn't hostile. Ultimately, the contract was agreed to and we moved on.

A renovation had been done on the cafeteria at our upper elementary school a few years prior. One day during lunch periods, the tubular ventilation ductwork broke free and fell, injuring some students and staff. Except for our board president, we all stayed away from the scene. The local district attorney investigated the occurrence and found no criminal wrongdoing on the districts part. Still, it isn't pleasant when something like that happens on your watch.

Most boards have committees. Our board had a few members who got elected to lead the district then didn't necessarily want to do so. I was tasked with heading 3 committees at one point or another. I stayed away from the athletic committee. My last 2 years had me heading up the Policy Committee and the Buildings and Grounds Committee. One of the big policy changes that came up had to do with Title IX reporting to the state. I led a number of meetings to address this and, with input from our booster groups, we amended the policy appropriately.

In my last 2 years on the board, we commissioned a feasibility study to determine how to best organize our district due to dwindling numbers of students. Our district declined by about 1000 students in a 10-year period and the state and a demographer indicated that it wasn't going to change any time soon. Decisions are sometimes made easier by events that occur. We had a fire occur in one of our primary schools. Part of our feasibility study said to reduce the number of buildings in our district by one or 2. We ultimately opted to build a new, larger building on the site and close one of the smaller schools.

The final major item I was involved with was an early bird contract for our teachers. Living through a strike was difficult for all in the community and we wanted to avoid it again. The negotiating teams were different on both sides this time (save for me) and the union president. We were able to accomplish a reasonable contract in 2 meetings. I left feeling pretty good about that since it extended any potential problems out by 5 years.

During all this I still went to work each day at the high school. I made a concerted effort to separate the 2 positions. I know people, (staff, administration and coaches) felt at times that I was looking over their shoulder. I never went to a board meeting and said to anyone, "I saw (person) doing such and such in the building." I did, however, always get an earful from our athletic director who was in the habit of pushing his agenda on me. My impression of him was that he was always in the coaches' corner when problems arose and he tended to assume that parents were the cause of problems more than anything else. It was nice to be able to speak freely with the building principal and from time to time we would chat. I kept our conversations on the educational side of things. We would discuss test scores and how to improve them as well as the changing educational environment. I learned a lot from him and still speak to him about education issues. Most students and parents had no idea I was a member of the school board. I was fine with that and really didn't want that to change as I was there to do a job, not spend time rubbing elbows.

My four-year term ended in December of 2015. I consider it a privilege and honor to have been able to serve my community. It isn't an easy thing to do considering the possibility that when a decision is made, you may be blamed. There is a lot of time and learning that goes into the job. It is an unpaid elected position. I have the "thank you" clock sitting on my desk at home as a reminder of my time there.

REFLECTION

I enjoyed my time in public service. I made many new acquaintances and learned a lot about politics and people. It is not something I would attempt again while in my contracted position. It was, at times, difficult to have conversations and debates with those in opposition to my ideas, knowing that at some point in the future those same people would be deciding on my employment. My health system did secure a new contract after my departure from the board. I remain in the position I have had for 25 years, and I hope to finish my career here.

Murder in the Bluegrass

Al Green, MEd, LAT, ATC, EMT

Key Terms

Post-traumatic Stress Disorder

As an athletic trainer, you are taught to be prepared for anything. You practice your skills regularly and you commit to increasing your knowledge through continuing education programs. There are some instances, however, where you have an event that you just cannot prepare for, an event that isn't written about in any textbook. An event that changes you and all around you.

True Story #34

It was a typical July weekend during the summer in Lexington, Kentucky. I was the head athletic trainer at the University of Kentucky and my wife, Sue, was the associate head athletic trainer. Sue went to her office at the E. J. Nutter Training Facility to catch up on a few things. Both of us provided care for the football team and even though it was a Saturday in the summer, the work never ended. Sue remembers sitting in her office overlooking the practice field and seeing a football player running all by himself. She said to herself, "On Monday, I need to congratulate him on earning a football scholarship for his senior season." Trent DiGuiro was a walk-on during his time at Kentucky so earning a scholarship was a major accomplishment. She also wanted to tell him how proud she was of him for working so hard to earn that scholarship. How many players come in on Saturday to run and work out by themselves? Sue never had that chance to praise Trent on his accomplishment.

That Saturday night, July 17, 1994, Trent DiGuiro was killed on his front pouch celebrating his twenty-first birthday. Surrounded by his teammates and friends, he died from being shot in the head by a high-powered rifle. No one at the party saw or heard anything prior to or after the shot. That moment forever changed the lives of Trent's family, friends, teammates, coaches, and athletic trainers.

The phone call came soon after the shooting. As usual, if the phone rang in the middle of the night in the Stanley-Green household, one of us answered while the other one got up and started getting dressed. We knew we were going to have to go somewhere to deal with a crisis that involved one of our athletes. Nothing could have prepared us for that call. All the players and friends who were at the party that night were taken to the Lexington Police Department for questioning. We immediately headed to the police station. On the way, we drove past the house were the shooting occurred. We saw a flurry of police activity as the crime scene units were searching for and gathering evidence. We went to the police station and met with the players and started putting the pieces of night together. We took the players back to the Nutter Center since the house was still off limits and to help try to make some sense of what had just happened. The players looked to us for answers. We are the fixers. We are the ones that make everything okay. We are there parents away from home. That night, all we could do was to hold them and be there for them. There was no fixing and no answers to give.

It was now close to 6 o' clock AM and time to put our catastrophic plan in motion. We had already notified the athletic director who would contact the university administration. Next it was time to notify the coaching staff. We called Coach Curry, the head coach, several times but he did not answer. We knew he had been out of town and he was supposed to return on Saturday night. It was now Sunday morning. The coaches started to arrive at Nutter to console the players as best they could. It was decided Sue and I would go to his house and leave him a note to call us as soon as he got home. This was precell phone days and no one was as accessible as today. It turned out a tree limb fell on the phone line and he had no service.

As we drove up, we saw lights on. We knew he was an early riser and to our surprise, he was home. Coach Curry's wife, Carolyn, answered the door delighted to see us. Sadly, Coach Curry knew that if Al and Sue arrived at his house uninvited at 6 o' clock, it was not a good thing. Coach Bill Curry is one of the most caring, kind, compassionate men that has ever coached a football team at any level. He and Carolyn were devastated with the news. His son, Billy Curry was good friends with Trent and was inconsolable. Coach Curry wanted to get to the players as soon as possible. He wanted to go by the house, Sue and I drove him directly to Trent's house which was close to campus.

When we arrived, some of the players were wandering around in a daze. The police had collected all the evidence they needed and on the porch, was the overstuffed brown chair where Trent had been sitting and a great deal of blood. The press was starting to gather so Coach Curry decided he didn't want them to see and film all the blood. I tried to get Coach to let me come back and clean it a little later. I am a volunteer firefighter and emergency medical technician, so I am very familiar with this type of scene and cleaning it up. Coach Curry needed to do this, so he, Sue, some of Trent's fellow offensive linemen, and I hosed, swept, mopped and cleaned Trent's blood that was spilled on that front porch. This was a surreal moment for us and a memory that wasn't easily erased by time. One thing that stood out to me was how the media recognized that this as a private moment and stopped filming. I know today that would not have happened.

The murder of Trent DiGuiro threw the entire football program into turmoil. There weren't any motives or suspects. Speculation grew almost immediately. Was Trent or other teammates involved in drugs, steroids, or gambling that could result in someone trying to retaliate? Was the killer going to strike again? It was very tense as we went into the 1994 football season. Many of the players were at the house when the murder happened and were greatly affected. As you looked into their eyes, the fear was apparent. Our team psychologist held debriefings with the players. Grief counselors were brought in. Without answers and motive, fear was a constant for our players. Many felt they were next. Many felt they were being followed, phone calls where the caller hung up or just didn't speak were received, a flat tire, anything was a sign that they were next. All who were there, and many who were not, were suffering from what today is known as post-traumatic stress disorder or PTSD. Many suffered from the classic symptoms of flashbacks, insomnia, nightmares, anger, irritability, always on guard and loss of interest in football and life. We would meet daily and talk to players trying to calm their fears or just be a sounding board for their feelings. Several were referred for counseling. Part of our job, besides being there and supporting them through this tough time, was to monitor the players and intervene when necessary.

Our cross-state rival, the University of Louisville, was our first opponent. The players came out fired up and took their anger, aggression, and fear out on Louisville. We won that very emotional game. After the game in the locker room, the players cried, rolled around on the floor, and agonized about the loss of their teammate. The football team did not win another game that season. The coaches tried everything. They were tough on them and practiced them harder and longer than usual. That didn't work so they took them to movies and provided extra food, snacks, and treats. They tried anything and everything to get them back on track. There were too many unanswered questions and raw emotions. A death threat against Coach Curry's family heightened everyone's fears. The season was over after that first game.

As an athletic trainer, the frustration was immense. You want to nurture everyone. You want to make it okay. You take care of everyone else, but at the same time you are grieving for the loss of one of your kids. There wasn't a motive, arrest, or even a suspect. Without answers, there wasn't any closure. For years everyone associated with the 1994 University of Kentucky football team were left wondering. This remains one of the most devastating and emotional times for both Sue and I. Trent was the second of 3 University of Kentucky athletes who died within a 2-year period.

The investigation into the murder of Trent DiGuiro went on for years. It was featured on several television shows including *America's Most Wanted*. Finally, after many years, there was a break in the case. A former girlfriend of the shooter came forward. She couldn't live with the guilt anymore. She was wired and got a taped confession. It was determined the murder occurred because the person who pulled the trigger thought Trent was having him blackballed from a fraternity. The sad reality was Trent was not there the night of the vote and had not blackballed him. The person was convicted and sentenced to 30 years. He spent only a few years in jail before he was released on a technicality. In an ironic twist, he was later injured in a car accident that left him a quadriplegic.

REFLECTION

When you pass your board of certification exam, you feel you can handle anything. You realize the fractures, dislocations, concussions, sprains and strains are the easy fixes. Sometimes you are faced with a crisis that there is no plan for, which is not taught in the classroom, one that will test you. This was a difficult time but, in a way, one that was also rewarding. Being there for athletes when they are scared and in pain is an honor and privilege. Later you reflect on it as a rewarding and memorable time in your career, a time you made a difference in people's lives and they made a difference in yours.

VOCATIONAL DISCERNMENT

Richard Ray, EdD, ATC

KEY TERMS

Vocation | Employment Setting | Job Satisfaction

How do many of us (especially when new to the profession) take the time to diligently and thoroughly discern our vocational fit with any of the many settings in which athletic trainers are commonly employed? With graduation, certification, and licensure within view on the horizon, perhaps we're too anxious to get a job instead of doing what we should to ensure that we get the job that's right for us. This is a story of one athletic trainer's decision to ignore his heart and how the limelight almost derailed a promising career as a result.

TRUE STORY #35

I came of age as an athletic trainer during a time when most of us were professionally educated in an apprenticeship model. We were college educated, of course, but what we knew about athletic training we learned by imitating those experienced practitioners who served as our mentors, guides, and informal teachers. The settings in which I apprenticed consisted exclusively of big time college and professional athletics. I attended a big 10 university and interned during 2 summers for a highly competitive National Football League team. While in college, I worked with national caliber football and ice hockey teams—teams that played in Rose Bowls and National Collegiate Athletic Association Division I championship games. I also worked (almost completely unsupervised) with my university's women's basketball team when Title IX of the Education Amendments Act was very new and the environment in which women participated in college athletics was very different than it is today. With the exception of the women on the basketball team, most of the athletes with whom I associated were looking toward careers as professional athletes. Why shouldn't I also set my athletic training ambitions on the highest level possible after graduation?

As my college graduation approached, and with my certification exam passed, I felt that I should attend graduate school for a Master's degree to give myself the best chance at the kind of high-level athletic training job I was confident was my destiny. Newly married, I selected a nearby university that would allow my wife and I to live in her hometown. I would also be able to finish graduate school in one year, an important consideration, as I was anxious to be finished with school and to make my mark on the world. The university where I pursued my graduate degree was (like my undergraduate alma mater) a big place that sponsored a competitive Division I athletic program. Though I requested the opportunity to work with one of the university's teams, the graduate program director assigned me to be the head athletic trainer across the street at the local Division III college. I was disappointed. The undergraduate-serving, liberal arts college was a setting unlike anything I'd known up to that point in my life. At first it seemed more like high school athletics than the professionalized sporting environments I'd experienced in college and during my summer National Football League internships. It was immediately evident that I would have very little in the way of money, supplies, or equipment in carrying out my responsibilities. Even the athletic training room was shabby and consisted of a small space with a concrete floor partitioned off from the rest of a visiting team locker room. I filled the whirlpool in the shower room and drained it through the door and onto the track. This was not what I imagined when I thought of myself as an athletic trainer.

With each relationship, and with each passing day, small college life began to enchant me. The athletes were certainly students first. They practiced hard and wanted to win, but were also very bright. They inquired about the physics of therapeutic ultrasound while undergoing treatment. They wondered about the physiology of inflammation and tissue healing during rehabilitation. They said "please" and "thank you" as a regular part of our daily interactions. The coaches were long-time, respected members of the college faculty. They sought my recommendations, listened carefully, and thanked me for my contributions. Not a week went past without someone asking how my graduate school classes were going. The president of the college knew my name. This was a place where I worked as hard as I had during my undergraduate years, but it was a place peopled with others who cared about me as part of a shared learning community. Even now, 40 years later, I can remember where I was when I said to myself, "I think I'd like to work at a place like this one day."

As my graduate program began to wind down and a serious job search moved into high gear, I found myself applying for every athletic training position advertised. In fact, I applied for about 80 positions. I applied for jobs for which I knew I was unqualified. I applied for jobs I knew I did not want. "Apply, apply, apply" was my daily mantra. Each day brought fresh letters of rejection and previously unknown levels of anxiety.

Persistence, patience, and good fortune eventually paid dividends and rewarded me with 3 job interviews, each of which resulted in an offer of employment. I had the choice of serving a large urban high school, a small Division III liberal arts college, or a large Division I university. The high school never seriously interested me for reasons that seemed obvious then but poorly discerned now. The liberal arts college might have captured my imagination, but the salary was so low that I couldn't imagine how I would eke out a living. When I asked the athletic director about the low salary, he responded unhelpfully by informing me that my wife could get a job someplace. The Division I university appealed to all of my instincts and most of my experiences. I'd be working with the nationally ranked men's basketball team as my primary assignment. I'd be traveling the country and the world while making terrific connections that would serve my career for many years to come. I'd be rubbing elbows with outstanding athletes who would soon be playing in the National Basketball Association. The money wasn't great, but as things turned out I came to learn that you don't need much money if you're hardly ever home to spend it. Master's degree in hand, my wife and I packed the U-Haul and headed to Big State University, where (we thought) the bright lights awaited.

The first couple of months at Big State University went well enough. The other members of the athletic training staff treated me well despite my big, untested ideas about how things could be improved. When I think back, I now realize that their patience with me was enormous. The only concern that lingered in the recesses of my mind was related to the basketball coach. He was a seasoned, successful competitor on the national stage (and at Big State University basketball was the big sport). Which made him the king of Big State University. His word, I would later learn, was law. The athletic trainer who had worked with his team prior to my arrival was a hall of famer who was so respected and so revered that he was the only person who could tell the acerbic basketball coach where to get off and get away with it. Tragically, this fellow suffered a massive cardiac arrest and died. While his untimely death provided an opportunity for me, it also proved to be just what the coach wanted, a chance to get his way with a fresh-faced, 23-year-old rookie athletic trainer who discovered that he was soon in over his head.

It didn't take long for the coach to assert his authority at my expense. Our disagreements started small and quickly grew to encompass fundamental issues of foundational principles for which neither of us was willing to compromise. Things came to a head early in my first season when one of the team's best players (who would go on to a 10-year National Basketball Association career) sprained his ankle in practice. I assisted him to the athletic training room, evaluated the injury, applied ice, and elevated his ankle. Then I went back to the gym to let the coach know the situation.

"Get him back out here," he instructed me.

"Coach, he can't walk," I replied.

"Didn't you hear me the first time? Get him back out here."

I walked back to the athletic training room in a state of shock and confusion. Wasn't the coach going to listen to and respect my opinions? Was he going to override my judgments about return-to-play for even the most clear-cut cases? I fitted the athlete with crutches and helped him back to the gym, where he stood on the sideline for 5 minutes before the coach snarled and kicked him out of practice.

I could barely sleep that night. Was this the kind of professional working relationship I would have to endure? I thought about how foreign the day's incident would have seemed at the liberal arts college I served during graduate school. I decided that it must just have been a misunderstanding, one I could clear up with a conversation the next day with the coach. When I went to see him in his office to voice my concerns about how the previous day's injury had been handled, he asked, "Do you want to help our team?" I assured him that I did, and that I was working 15-hour days trying to do so. "If you want to help our team, just do whatever I tell you to do," he told me without looking up from the newspaper he was reading. "You can leave now," he said as a way of concluding our meeting.

Did I mention that I was young, impetuous, and sure that I had all the answers? Well, I was. And I knew that I could not do what the coach expected me to do. So I went to the athletic director, told him the story, and asked for his advice. He assured me that the coach's bark was worse than his bite, counseled me to work with him and in his system, and that things would eventually be alright. The following morning the coach stormed into the athletic training room and asked me if I had gone to the athletic director. When I confirmed that I had done so, he told me I was fired. I informed him that I worked for the head athletic trainer and that when he told me I was fired I'd be fired. "Well I don't want you anywhere near my team," he growled. "You're fired from basketball." I responded to this insult by asking which undergraduate athletic training student he wanted to entrust the health of his team to when it traveled to the big rivalry game in 2 days. "Anyone but you," was his response.

Two months into my first job, and I was a failure.

While the next couple of days were the worst of my professional life, things did eventually cool down. Trembling with fear, I got on the bus 2 days later and was greeted by a cold stare from the coach, but he didn't kick me off. In fact, he never really bothered me after that. Perhaps he developed some modest level of respect for me once he learned that I was willing to stick up for myself. Still, I knew I was in the wrong place. I knew I should have listened to my heart and employed my gifts in the Division III liberal arts college where they would have been more sincerely appreciated. I restarted my job search that weekend. It would take me another 18 months, but eventually I found a job in a liberal arts college that shares my values. It has served as a place to incubate my personal and professional growth for nearly 4 decades.

Reflection

The writer and theologian Frederick Buechner famously informs us that, "Vocation is the place where our deep gladness meets the world's deep need." Had I more carefully discerned my own set of talents during my days as a student and had I considered how and in what ways my values aligned (or not) with the dominant athletic ethos of big time university sports, I could have avoided the painful lessons of my first job. I knew that my experience in the liberal arts college during graduate school filled me in ways that nothing else had up to that point. Still, I looked away, blinded by what I thought were the bright lights. Ultimately, I came to learn that while I loved being an athletic trainer, I neither needed nor wanted the bright lights. I did not need the bright lights to cultivate the kind of relationships that time, wisdom, and experience came to teach me were most available in settings where athletics was a treasured adjunct to a well-rounded education and not the main event that they so often were at Big State University. I wish someone, one of my teachers perhaps, had engaged me in a process of vocational discernment and forced me through disciplined thinking to articulate my deeply held values and to think about how those values might inform a host of decisions, including the decision about how and where to employ my gifts. In some ways, I'm glad I had the 2 years at Big State University, but I escaped to the sunlit uplands of the place I truly belonged only after paying a significant emotional price. Did it have to be so?

FINANCIAL DISCLOSURES

Dr. Adam Annaccone has not disclosed any relevant financial relationships.

Dr. Morgan Cooper Bagley has not disclosed any relevant financial relationships.

Robert O. Blanc has no financial or proprietary interest in the materials presented herein.

Richard Burr has no financial or proprietary interest in the materials presented herein.

Dr. Paul A. Cacolice has no financial or proprietary interest in the materials presented herein.

Dr. Douglas Casa has received grant/research/clinical trial support from Mission; Welkins; General Electric; Quest; CamelBak; National Football League; Kestrel; One Beat, Heartsmart.com, Brainscope, WHOOP, National Athletic Trainers' Association, Polar, Gatorade; Danone; Timex; University of North Carolina; US Air Force; US Army (preventing sudden death in sport, heat stroke; thermoregulation; hydration [cooling products, hydration products, wearable technology]). He is a consultant for/on the advisory board of Quest, (biomarkers) Sports Innovation Labs, Clif Bar. He has been an expert witness on legal cases (heat stroke, exertional sickening, dehydration), and he receives royalties from Jones and Bartlett, Springer, Lippincott Williams & Wilkins publishers.

Robert J. Casmus has not disclosed any relevant financial relationships.

Dr. James Cerullo has no financial or proprietary interest in the materials presented herein.

Dr. Kevin Conley has not disclosed any relevant financial relationships.

Larry Cooper has not disclosed any relevant financial relationships.

Bill Couts has not disclosed any relevant financial relationships.

Tim Dunlavey has not disclosed any relevant financial relationships.

Dr. Francis Feld has no financial or proprietary interest in the materials presented herein.

Tim Giel has not disclosed any relevant financial relationships.

Dr. Keith M. Gorse has no financial or proprietary interest in the materials presented herein.

Al Green has not disclosed any relevant financial relationships.

Michael Hanley has not disclosed any relevant financial relationships.

Dr. Timothy J. Henry has no financial or proprietary interest in the materials presented herein.

Dr. Valerie Herzog has no financial or proprietary interest in the materials presented herein.

Dr. Peggy A. Houglum has no financial or proprietary interest in the materials presented herein.

Ryan Johnson has no financial or proprietary interest in the materials presented herein.

Kyle Johnston has not disclosed any relevant financial relationships.

Dr. Blake LeBlanc has not disclosed any relevant financial relationships.

Dr. Sarah Manspeaker has not disclosed any relevant financial relationships.

Kate McCartney has not disclosed any relevant financial relationships.

Ryan McGovern has not disclosed any relevant financial relationships.

Randy McGuire has no financial or proprietary interest in the materials presented herein.

Dr. David H. Perrin has no financial or proprietary interest in the materials presented herein.

Marirose Radelet has not disclosed any relevant financial relationships.

Dr. Richard Ray is the author of a text published by Human Kinetics.

Gaetano Sanchioli has not disclosed any relevant financial relationships.

Jeff Shields has not disclosed any relevant financial relationships.

Dr. Rebecca L. Stearns is an employee for the Korey Stringer Institute at the University of Connecticut and an Editor for book published by Jones and Bartlett Publishers.

Dr. Giampietro L. Vairo has not disclosed any relevant financial relationships.

Sam Zuege has no financial or proprietary interest in the materials presented herein.

Mary Mundrane-Zweiacher has not disclosed any relevant financial relationships.

INDEX